Central Venous Access

Central Venous Access

Editor

Charles E. Ray, Jr., M.D.

Chief, Interventional Radiology
Denver Health Medical Center
Associate Professor of Radiology
University of Colorado Health Sciences Center
Denver, Colorado

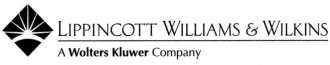

LIPPINCOTT WILLIAMS & WILKINS
A **Wolters Kluwer** Company
Philadelphia · Baltimore · New York · London
Buenos Aires · Hong Kong · Sydney · Tokyo

Acquisitions Editor: Beth K. Barry
Developmental Editor: Selina M. Bush
Supervising Editor: Steven P. Martin
Production Editor: Janet Domingo, Compset, Inc.
Manufacturing Manager: Tim Reynolds
Cover Designer: Mark Lerner
Compositor: Compset, Inc.
Printer: Maple Press

© 2001 by LIPPINCOTT WILLIAMS & WILKINS
530 Walnut Street
Philadelphia, PA 19106 USA
LWW.com

Printed in the USA

Library of Congress Cataloging-in-Publication Data
Central venous access / editor, Charles E. Ray, Jr.
   p. ; cm.
Includes bibliographical references and index.
  ISBN 0-7817-2905-X (hardcover : alk. paper)
  1. Blood-vessels—Cutdown. 2. Intravenous catheterization. 3. Arteriovenous shunts, Surgical.
  [DNLM: 1. Catheterization, Central Venous—methods. 2. Catheterization, Central Venous—instrumentation. 3. Catheters, Indwelling. WB 26 C397 2001] I. Ray, Charles E.
  RD 598.5 .C45 2001
  617.4'14—dc21

2001034416

Care has been taken to confirm the accuracy of the information presented and to describe generally accepted practices. However, the authors, editors, and publisher are not responsible for errors or omissions or for any consequences from application of the information in this book and make no warranty, expressed or implied, with respect to the currency, completeness, or accuracy of the contents of the publication. Application of this information in a particular situation remains the professional responsibility of the practitioner.

The authors, editors, and publisher have exerted every effort to ensure that drug selection and dosage set forth in this text are in accordance with current recommendations and practice at the time of publication. However, in view of ongoing research, changes in government regulations, and the constant flow of information relating to drug therapy and drug reactions, the reader is urged to check the package insert for each drug for any change in indications and dosage and for added warnings and precautions. This is particularly important when the recommended agent is a new or infrequently employed drug.

Some drugs and medical devices in this publication have Food and Drug Administration (FDA) clearance for limited use in restricted research settings. It is the responsibility of the health care provider to ascertain the FDA status of each drug or device planned for use in their clinical practice.

10 9 8 7 6 5 4 3 2 1

DEDICATION

To my most influential teachers:
Bradford Rence, Ph.D., (Appleton),
for introducing me to the scientific method;
William Bremer, Ph.D., (Appleton), for educating me that
acquiring knowledge in any form is a noble and definitive goal;
W. Franklin Hughes, Ph.D., (Chicago), for allowing me
to understand the challenges facing the medical researcher;
John Kaufman, M.D., (Portland), for teaching me
by example that we are physicians first, investigators second;
and my parents, wife, and daughter, for teaching me
the most valuable lessons along the way.

Contents

Contributing Authors ix

Preface xi

Acknowledgements xiii

1. Building a Central Venous Access Device Service 1

2. Venous Anatomy 9

3. Imaging Guidance for Central Venous Access 19

4. Preprocedural Assessment 49

5. Short- and Intermediate-Term Central Venous Catheters 57

6. Implantable Port Devices 63

7. Tunneled Catheters 73

8. Hemodialysis Access 87

9. Peripherally Inserted Central Catheters 95

10. Postprocedure Care of Venous Access Devices 105

11. Central Venous Access Device Placement in Pediatric Patients 115

12. Alternative Routes of Central Venous Catheter Placement 129

13. Central Venous Access: A Cost Analysis 145

14. Complications of Central Venous Access Devices 151

    Subject Index 165

Contributing Authors

Iftikhar Ahmad, M.D.   *Clinical Assistant Professor, Department of Radiology, Indiana University Medical Centre, Indianapolis, Indiana*

Chieh-Min Fan, M.D.   *Instructor, Division of Vascular Radiology, Harvard Medical School; Assistant Radiologist, Department of Radiology, Massachusetts General Hospital, Boston, Massachusetts*

Jan Durham, M.D.   *Associate Professor, Department of Interventional Radiology, University of Colorado Health Sciences Center, Denver, Colorado*

Atul K. Gupta, M.D.   *Assistant Professor, Department of Radiology, State University of New York at Buffalo School of Medicine; Director of Angiography and Interventional Radiology, Department of Radiology, Roswell Park Cancer Institute, Buffalo, New York*

Roger K. Harned II, M.D.   *Assistant Professor, Department of Radiology, University of Colorado Health Sciences Center; Pediatric Radiologist, Department of Radiology, The Children's Hospital, Denver, Colorado*

John A. Kaufman, M.D.   *Professor, Dotter Interventional Institute, Portland, Oregon*

Tom B. Kinney, M.D.   *Assistant Professor, Department of Vascular and Interventional Radiology, University of California Medical Center, San Diego, California*

Jan Namyslowski, M.D.   *Assistant Professor, Department of Radiology, Indiana University School of Medicine, University Hospital, Indianapolis, Indiana*

Pamela D. Paplham, N.P.   *Family Nurse Practitioner, Department of Medical Oncology, Roswell Park Cancer Institute, Buffalo, New York*

Charles E. Ray, Jr., M.D.   *Chief, Division of Interventional Radiology, Denver Health Medical Center; Associate Professor of Radiology, University of Colorado Health Sciences Center, Denver, Colorado*

Guido M. Scatorchia, M.D.   *Assistant Professor, Department of Radiology, University of Colorado Health Sciences Center; Division of Interventional Radiology, Denver Health Medical Center, Denver, Colorado*

James H. Turner, M.D.   *Assistant Professor, Department of Radiology, University of Colorado Health Sciences Center; Interventional Radiologist, Division of Interventional Radiology, Denver Health Medical Center, Denver, Colorado*

Preface

It wasn't long ago that interventional radiologic procedures were nonexistent. As interventional procedures have evolved, so too has the role of the interventionalist. Diagnostic angiography was the initial duty of the interventionalist; indeed, even today (including at the editor's own institution), many interventional procedure films are housed in jackets containing simply the title, *Angio*. Over the years, however, interventional radiology has developed into a true clinical specialty, complete with consults, admitting services, and seemingly endless paperwork!

Over the years, many new procedures have either been dreamed up by the radiologic society (e.g., transjugular intrahepatic portosystem shunts [TIPS] and embolization procedures) or have been assumed by radiologists from other fields. Central venous access device (CVAD) placement belongs in the latter category. Initially falling under the auspices of surgeons, radiologists realized that the combination of needle/guidewire/catheters was uniquely suited to their skills. Add to these basic tools the role of imaging guidance, and the match of CVAD and radiology was complete.

It is perhaps because of this ever-changing role that radiologists feel under pressure, even at times threatened, to continue to explore new opportunities within the medical field. Whether this assertive approach is met with open arms or obstacles is largely a function of the individual radiologist's practice setting. Regardless of the political environment, however, the best stance for anyone to take is the practice of sound, solid medicine. Although doing so does not guarantee a booming interventional practice, <u>not</u> doing so assures failure.

It was for this reason that the following book was written. This text is meant to be a guide for developing and maintaining a solid CVAD practice. It is not intended to be a definitive, extensive tome on one aspect of interventional practice. Rather, it is hoped that individuals on the threshold of developing a CVAD practice will find both the theoretical and practical information contained herein helpful to the development of their own CVAD service.

Acknowledgments

The editor wishes to thank the following individuals for their contributions to this book: all of the contributing authors, without whose selfless and timely work this text undoubtedly could not have been completed; Selina Bush and Beth Barry at Lippincott Williams & Wilkins, without whose guidance this project would have proved to be unattainable; and Stacy Erickson, whose artwork has adorned not just the pages of this volume but numerous other projects as well.

Central Venous Access

Central Venous Access
Edited by Charles E. Ray, Jr.
Lippincott Williams & Wilkins, Philadelphia © 2001.

1

Building a Central Venous Access Device Service

Charles E. Ray, Jr., MD

Denver Health Medical Center;
University of Colorado Health Sciences Center, Denver, Colorado 80204

Central venous access devices (VAD) are increasingly being placed by radiologists; many interventional radiology (IR) groups now devote greater than half of their time or half of their caseload to VAD placement. The advantages of radiologic placement of VADs are numerous (Table 1.1). Although VAD placement may eventually become overwhelming in some settings, initiating a service often proves difficult due to a variety of factors: turf battles with other clinical services, hospital privileges, lack of formal training in the procedures, and the preconceived notions of a "radiologist's role" all pose potential roadblocks to developing a successful line service. The purpose of this chapter is to provide practical guidelines to aid in the development of a VAD service, and to suggest methods by which to initiate a VAD service and to keep the service successful in the long term.

ROLE OF THE RADIOLOGIST

Interventional radiologists truly are unique specialists within the field of medicine. Interventionalists are usually members of a diagnostic radiology department, and as such are usually considered by referring physicians as radiologists first and interventionalists second. This affiliation is particularly strong in the private sector, where IR physicians might go from performing an arteriogram to doing a barium study, from performing an angioplasty to reading a stack of mammograms. Referring physicians un-

derstandably might be confused as to the role of IR within the radiology department. Adding to the confusion is the fact that most interventionalists require the preprocedure evaluation of a patient to be performed by the referring clinical service. As procedure-oriented physicians, interventionalists are unique in that way—all other invasive physicians (e.g., surgeons, gastroenterologists, anesthesiologists, etc.) receive a consult and then assess the patient directly. It seems that only in IR do we not only expect physicians to refer patients to us, but we expect the uninteresting work such as admission orders and scheduling forms to be completed by the individual requesting the consult. This arrangement is a poor enough setup in an academic hospital, where residents and fellows abound, but in the private sector, referring physicians typically want no part of the consultant who makes more rather than less work for the referring doctor. Interventionalists, therefore, must recognize the need for a paradigm shift away from being the "doctor's doctor" into more of an active, patient-oriented, consulting clinician's role. Assuming the new role for the IR physician is an essential step, and nowhere is it more important than in the development of a VAD service.

Certain criteria are expected of consultants, which may be described as the three "abilities" of a successful consultant. In descending order of importance, the abilities required of consultants are *availability, amiability,* and *ability.* When functioning as diagnostic radiologists,

TABLE 1.1. *Advantages to radically-placed VAD*

More safe and successful than surgically placed VAD (1–10)

Significant cost-savings (16–18)

Ability to place VAD in via alternative approaches in patients with limited access (11–15)

Use of imaging guidance to decrease the risk of catheter malposition

Lower burden on operating room

More timely placement of VAD (typically within 24 hours)

VAD, venous access device.

interventionalists are familiar with being amiable and, hopefully, able consultants. It comes as no surprise, however, that many of our medical colleagues in other specialties frequently question the availability of radiologists during off-hours. Dealing with this preconceived notion of individuals who work "banker's hours" makes the development of any interventional service, including a VAD service, difficult. Availability, therefore, is a key component in the development of a VAD service. It is a short-lived service that tries to run from 8 a.m. to 5 p.m., and one that will not be well-received by our referring physicians.

In academic centers, the issue of availability might be easier to address than in the private sector. In teaching hospitals, it is not unreasonable to defer nonemergent cases to the morning shift, whereas emergency venous access (temporary central access, Swan-Ganz catheters) may be referred to the in-house surgical service. When following this algorithm, rarely is one called upon to place a VAD radiologically in the middle of the night. Care must be taken, however, not to deny performing a procedure out of hand simply because of the time of day. A rule of thumb that I use is to have the surgical service initially attempt the line placement at the patient's bedside; in the event of a failed attempt, the line is placed under radiologic guidance, regardless of the hour. Once referring physicians realize that you as a consultant are indeed willing to assist with difficult cases, the potential for conflict diminishes appreciably.

The concept of availability in the private setting may be significantly different from that seen in academic centers. Not only may in-hospital surgeons be lacking, but the dearth of in-house radiology residents or fellows may further complicate matters. Unfortunately, a general rule of thumb for private settings is not realistic; each individual situation depends in large part on already established relationships with referring services, the size of the radiology group (e.g., individuals who take IR calls every night vs. those who take them on a less frequent basis), and the commitment and availability of support staff.

In any setting, academic or private, the availability of the IR physician as a consultant is mandatory. Although actual placement of devices might be deferred until normal working hours, one must expect off-hour questions concerning not just placement of VADs but management issues regarding their care. Questions regarding the type of device to place, postprocedure care of the device, and how to best deal with VAD-related complications are commonly asked at any hour. Any physician placing such devices must be available (and amiable) if and when such questions arise.

Placing the VAD is only one component of running a VAD service. In addition to placement of the device, the radiologist must be willing and able to assume the role of manager of patients in whom VAD are placed. The position also requires the individual to become familiar with currently available VADs, and when each device should be placed. Acting as a consultant for routine postprocedure care is also vital, and typically is addressed best through the nursing staff caring for the patient. Finally, being familiar with VAD complications, and the treatment of such complications, is also paramount. As stated earlier, most referring physicians could not care less who places the device in their patients—until something goes wrong. These issues (e.g., VAD-related complications) are further discussed in a later chapter.

INITIATING A VAD SERVICE

The first step in developing a successful VAD service is in properly initiating the service. Although intuitive, the initial phase of service development typically proves the most challenging and time consuming. In addition, many hours may be spent in the initial development phase without any immediate positive outcome; it may take months literally from the time of initiating the service to receiving the first consultation for a line placement.

One rule of thumb before initiating a line service is to be certain that the IR section placing the device is ready to start accepting patients for these procedures. It should not be assumed that a "fully stocked" angiography suite is ready to assume the added responsibility for VAD patients. Many VAD-specific issues should be addressed before the first procedure is performed.

Angiography Suite

In the best of all circumstances, any angiography suite in which lines will be placed will be operating room (OR) compatible. In general terms, OR-compatible rooms will possess a reverse ventilation system that circulates air far more frequently than a standard ventilation system; a dedicated scrub sink that is isolated from the main operating room; nonporous ceiling and floor tiles; and stainless-steel cabinets. In the era of venous access and stent graft procedures, most newly constructed angiography suites will be OR compatible (within the limits of the institution). If, however, an OR compatible room is neither available nor planned, any room with fluoroscopic equipment may be adequate for line placement. The literature is replete with outcomes studies that demonstrate no significant increase in infection rates for lines placed in the radiology department when compared with surgically placed lines in the operating suite (1–10).

Catheters and Guidewires

Depending on the devices being placed, standard or stock angiography equipment may be adequate to start a VAD service with a few notable additions.

Short guidewires (i.e., <60 cm in length) offer a great advantage over standard-length wires during VAD placement. If a standard 145- or 150-cm guidewire is used, it either must be advanced far into the venous system (e.g., into the iliac vein from a jugular approach), or a significant amount of wire will remain outside of the patient. In the latter circumstance, the large amount of wire outside the patient will be more difficult to control and, most importantly, can become contaminated during catheter or guidewire exchanges. With angiography or other commonly performed IR procedures, guidewire contamination is no great issue; with venous access, particularly when placing implantable or tunneled devices, contamination is an extremely important event that may preclude completion of the procedure or may cause increased infectious complications over the long run. Other additional guidewires, such as long, thin wires (e.g., 180 cm length, 0.018 inch diameter), may be needed when placing VADs such as peripherally inserted central catheters (PICC) or central Hohn catheters. Finally, because many of these catheters are blunt tipped or closed at their tip (Groshong tip catheters), standard over-the-wire technique may not be adequate in placing the catheters through the skin or subcutaneous tissues. Catheters may be difficult or impossible to advance over a wire, and *peel-away sheaths* may need to be placed in order to advance the catheters into or within the vein. For an active VAD service, it is necessary to stock multiple sheath sizes and lengths, typically varying from 4 to 14 French in diameter and 10 to 30 cm in length.

Microaccess systems consist of a 21-gauge needle, a short 0.018 inch diameter guidewire, and a coaxial 5–3 Fr dilator system (Cook, Inc., Bloomington, IN, U.S.A.). Microaccess systems allow puncture of the vessel with a small-gauge needle, and placement of a 5-Fr dilator capable of accepting a 0.038-inch guidewire, by adding two additional steps when compared with puncture using a standard 18-gauge needle. By performing the puncture with a thinner needle, accidental puncture of adjacent structures during venipuncture (e.g., artery, pleural surface) should result in a lesser complication than performing the same puncture using a larger gauge needle. Using the microaccess system is easily learned, adds minimally to the time of a procedure, and usually adds little cost to the procedure (typically $20–$30 per microaccess system). The main drawback to using the microaccess system is that it can be difficult to visualize the 21-gauge needle via ultrasonography. Tips for better needle visualization include roughing the needle tip with a scalpel in order to produce more accoustic reflectors; continuously bouncing the needle to and fro during advancement to visualize under ultrasonography the point of maximum tissue displacement (representing the tissue just distal to the needle tip); or purchasing a system with an accoustically visible needle tip.

Angiography Table

The arrangement of the table may differ significantly from the setup typically used in angiographic or drainage procedures. A list of items on the table for VAD placement at my institution is provided in Table 1.2.

Unlike angiography, the table used for placement of a VAD should be completely separate from the preparation table used for scrubbing the patient prior to the procedure. This practice is particularly important when placing an implantable or tunneled device. In addition, the in-

TABLE 1.2. *Items included on angiography table for VAD placement*

---

4 × 4 inch gauze (×20)
Syringes (×4)
   20 mL, Luerlock, labeled for lidocaine
   10 mL, slip-tip or Luerlock, used for needle
      aspiration during initial venous access
   10 mL (×2), slip-tip or Luerlock, used for catheter
      flushes, heparin flushes, etc.
Needles
   18-gauge, to draw lidocaine and/or sodium
      bicarbonate from single use vial or bottle
   25-gauge, for lidocaine administration
Curved Kelly clamp
Needle driver
Suture material (2-0 silk, 2-0 prolene, and/or 4-0
   vicryl)
Bowls (×2) for saline and discard OR closed syringe
   flush system.
No. 11 scalpel
No. 15 scalpel (for implantable port systems)
Microaccess system

---

dividual who sets up the operating table should don hat, mask, and gown and undergo a full surgical scrub before approaching the table. It makes no sense to have all of the operators undergo a surgical scrub, only to have the individual setting up the table be unmasked, ungowned, or unsterile.

Sterile Patient Preparation

Many different protocols can be used for sterile patient preparation; the number of different types of preparations for patients is almost as great as the number of operators. At my institution, the patients are prepared according to Table 1.3.

In addition to sterile patient preparation, each individual of the operating team must undergo a complete surgical scrub prior to donning gloves and gown. Hats and masks also must be worn by all members of the operating team. In addition, the individual who is to be responsible for draping the patient prior to the procedure should wear an extra set of gloves that can be removed between draping the patient and starting the procedure in case of any occult decontamination during the draping procedure. Gross contamination (e.g., accidentally touching an unprepared portion of the patient) requires a complete rescrub by the operator.

The above issues all represent deviations from the norm of work performed in an angiography section. It behooves the IR physician to be certain that all of the above issues are in order before attempting to initiate a line service; perhaps nothing will assure failure of a new technique more quickly than not having the correct equipment or personnel when the first referral arrives.

Scheduling Patients for VAD Placement

In remembering the importance of assuming a consultant's role, certain changes should be considered in the way in which patients are scheduled for VAD placements that may aid in the development of a line service.

TABLE 1.3. *Sterile surgical preparation*

1. Place hat and mask on the patient; the person performing the preparation should also wear a hat and mask.
2. Remove clothing and jewelry from a wide area around the operative field. For jugular and axillary/subclavian punctures, the prepared field should include from just below the ear to below the nipple line, from mid-axillary line to the sternum.
3. Administer Betadine scrub to the entire prepared field.
4. Repeat Betadine scrub.
5. Administer Betadine solution to the entire prepared field.
6. Repeat Betadine solution.
7. Cover the prepared area with a sterile towel.

The individual providing the above service should now break scrub and no longer be involved with the patient preparation.

8. If a prepared area is in danger of coming into contact with a nonsterile item (e.g., the prepared neck and underlying bedsheets or pillows), a sterile towel should be "scrunched" into the area to provide sterile protection.
9. Place folded towels or fenestrated sheet over operative field.
10. Remove top layer of gloves before proceeding to the procedure.

Referring physicians are accustomed to requesting radiology examinations via a subordinate; often these requests are written as orders in the patient's chart, and passed on either via a phone call or computer input by a nursing station clerk. Rather than accept requests in such a manner, it is my policy to require a physician-to-physician discussion prior to scheduling any VAD placement. The reasons for this requirement are not petty or insignificant. First, by assuring physician-to-physician contact, the referring physician begins to think of the IR physician as more of a consultant, distinct perhaps from his or her diagnostic radiology colleagues. Second, the referring physician often can be given a specific time frame in which the VAD can be placed, which is correctly perceived as a more complete referral than one given second-hand through clerical staff. Third, and perhaps most important, the IR physician can use the initial phone call to discuss the patient with the referring physician—to suggest which VAD is most appropriately used for any particular patient, to request more clinical information from the referring physician, and to assume a more active role in the patient's care than simply being the "line doctor." And although it may be difficult logistically to maintain the practice of discussions prior to each

case, it is an especially good procedure to implement at the early stages of service development.

PATIENT RECRUITMENT

Once the initial stage has been set, when the angiography suite and support staff are in line and ready to begin a VAD service, the question of how to best recruit patients arises. The specifics of recruiting patients depend entirely on the clinical, economic, and political implications of starting a line service in one's own hospital. Most frequently, interventionalists do not "recruit" patients on their own, but rather accept referrals from other physicians. In the best of all worlds, the IR physician fills a void within a particular hospital's practice setting; in most instances, however, the interventional VAD service instead competes directly with an already established service within the hospital. Other services (e.g., surgery) might find this competition threatening, causing a rift between the IR and surgical departments. How, then, to start a VAD-service without upsetting the political balance within an institution?

One method by which to initiate a VAD service is to offer radiologically guided placement of VADs in patients who have undergone an attempt at surgical placement of a catheter and failed, or to accept patients whom the surgeons do not wish to accept. Such patients would include obese patients, patients who have had previous VAD placements and may have symptomatic or occult venous stenoses or occlusions, patients with uncorrectable coagulopathies, or patients who may be difficult to manage intraprocedurally due to medical or psychological problems (11–15). Unfortunately, by assuming this strategy one is attempting to build a service with the most difficult patient population. One must be certain not to sabotage the service at the outset due to accepting the responsibility for this patient population, but success with this limited group of patients, and a willingness to attempt line placement for them, typically leads to a broadened referral base in the future.

A second way by which inroads may be made to initiating a VAD service is by placing devices that may not be available through other services. In other words, if the surgical service is able and willing to place implantable ports but not tunneled catheters, the most politically sound way to increase patient load might be by offering tunneled lines first, followed by other types of VAD in the future. In addition, if one's institution has PICC nurses available, but no other services are placing central intermediate care devices (e.g., Hohn catheters), the IR VAD service may be initiated by offering placement of those catheters.

If direct competition between the radiology and surgical services is unavoidable or irrelevant, then approaching other medical services in the hospital directly may be the most direct route to obtaining patients for VAD placements. Certain medical departments are usually the most active in terms of requesting VAD placements from the surgical service; these medical services typically include hematology/oncology, nephrology, critical care medicine, and infectious diseases. In approaching these services, one must remember that these potential referring physicians typically could not care less who places the VAD in their patient, as long as it is done safely and in a timely fashion. During the initial contact phases, presenting the services with literature regarding the safety of

radiologic placement of VAD may prove helpful; in addition, many references are available, indicating the cost effectiveness of radiologic placement of such devices (16–18). Other methods by which to approach potential referring services include offering to present a conference on VAD placement and care; providing in-services to the referring physicians and nurses regarding postprocedure care of VADs (most catheter company representatives would jump at the chance to be involved with such an educational exercise); and providing educational materials regarding VADs, such as when to place what device, or postprocedure catheter care algorithms. Again, the importance of providing a safe and timely service must be stressed.

EDUCATION OF THE RADIOLOGIST

One potential difficulty in establishing a VAD service is in the education or training of the physicians placing the devices. In reality, this issue is minor. Between general radiology conferences and interventional conferences, many educational opportunities exist for beginning or advanced VAD placement courses. Hands-on workshops, such as those presented yearly at the Society of Cardiovascular and Interventional Radiology annual meeting, are particularly helpful. In addition to presenting technical expertise, issues such as postprocedure care and recognizing and treating catheter-related complications are usually discussed.

In addition to such formal education pursued at conferences, practical education through mentoring is advantageous. In most large communities, there currently are radiologists placing VADs. Time spent with such physicians, even if in just an observatory role, may prove helpful in understanding the nuances of VAD placement. If necessary, minifellowships (e.g., a week or two) in interventional radiology are given by many of the larger medical centers; at all of these centers, VAD placement will be one of the major topics covered.

Regardless of the educational tack taken, it is imperative to document ALL forms of education. Without appropriate documentation, obtaining hospital privileges or convincing consulting physicians to refer patients may prove exceedingly difficult.

CONCLUSIONS

Many hurdles must be overcome during the initial stages of the development of a VAD service. Preconceived notions of the role of a radiologist, time-consuming processes such as obtaining hospital privileges or educating oneself prior to starting a service, being certain everything is in order prior to accepting the first patient, and dealing with "turf" battles with competing clinical services all represent obstacles in the development of a successful service. Most importantly, however, one must be willing to assume the role of primary provider for such patients and their devices. By following a few simple rules, initiating a VAD service is relatively straightforward and typically proves very fruitful for the IR service.

REFERENCES

1. Damascelli B, Patelli G, Frigerio LF, et al. Placement of long-term central venous catheters in outpatients: study of 134 patients over 24,596 catheter days. *AJR* 1997;168:1235–1239.
2. Shetty PC, Mody M, Kaston D, et al. Outcome of 350 implanted chest ports placed by interventional radiologists. *J Vasc Intervent Radiol* 1997;8:991–995.
3. Trerotola SO, Johnson MS, Harris VJ, et al. Outcome of tunneled hemodialysis catheters placed via the right internal jugular vein by interventional radiologists. *Radiology* 1997;203:489–495.
4. Kaufman JA, Salamipour H, Geller SC, et al. Long-term outcomes of radiologically placed arm ports. *Radiology* 1996;201:725–730.
5. Chait PG, Ingram J, Phillips-Gordon C, et al. PICCs in infants and children. *Radiology* 1995;197:775–778.
6. Openshaw KL, Picus D, Hicks ME, et al. Interventional radiologic placement of Hohn central venous catheters: results and complications in 100 consecutive patients. *J Vasc Intervent Radiol* 1994;5:111–115.
7. Cardella JF, Fox PS, Lawler JB. Interventional radiologic placement of PICCs. *J Vasc Intervent Radiol* 1993;4:653–660.
8. Denny DF. Placement and management of long-term central venous access catheters and ports. *AJR* 1993; 161:385–393.
9. Hull JE, Hunter CS, Luiken GA. The Groshong catheter: initial experience and early results of imaging-guided placement. *Radiology* 1992;185:803–807.
10. Gray RR. Radiologic placement of indwelling central venous lines for dialysis, TPN and chemotherapy. *J Intervent Radiol* 1991;6:133–144.
11. Patel NH. Alternate approaches to central venous access. *Semin Intervent Radiol* 1998;15:325–333.
12. Bennet JD, Papadouris D, Rankin RN, et al. Percutaneous inferior vena caval approach for long-term central venous access. *J Vasc Intervent Radiol* 1997;8: 851–855.
13. Kaufman JA, Greenfield AJ, Fitzpatrick GF. Transhepatic cannulation of the inferior vena cava. *J Vasc Intervent Radiol* 1991;2:331–334.
14. Meranze SG, McLean GK, Stein EJ, et al. Catheter placement in the azygous system: an unusual approach to venous access. *AJR* 1985;144:1075–1076.
15. Kaufman JA, Kazanjian SA, Rivitz SM, et al. Long-term central venous catheterization in patients with limited access. *AJR* 1996;167:1327–1333.
16. Noh HM, Kaufman JA, Fan CM, et al. Radiological approach to central venous catheters: cost analysis. *Semin Intervent Radiol* 1998;15:335–340.
17. Neuman ML, Murphy BD, Rosen MP. Bedside placement of peripherally inserted central catheters: a cost-effectiveness analysis. *Radiology* 1998;206:423–428.
18. Fan CM, Kaufman JA, Mason R, et al. Comparison of the cost of radiologic versus surgical placement of chest ports in outpatients. *Radiology* 1998;205:345.

Central Venous Access
Edited by Charles E. Ray, Jr.
Lippincott Williams & Wilkins, Philadelphia © 2001.

2

Venous Anatomy

Charles E. Ray, Jr., MD

Denver Health Medical Center;
University of Colorado Health Sciences Center, Denver, Colorado 80204

Catheters have been placed into the venous system of humans for almost 100 years (1). Central venous catheter placements have evolved over time; initially used for temporary or short-term access, such as a single dose of antibiotics via a peripherally accessed vein, longer term venous access became clinically possible with the advent of silastic, tunneled catheters (2). Since those sentinel descriptions, central venous access (CVA) procedures have continued to grow, as have the indications for placement of such devices. In part because of the increased use of CVA devices, many patients have had multiple devices placed over time, each carrying the risks inherent with such procedures (e.g., infection, venous thrombosis). Because many patients therefore do not present with "virgin" venous systems, the importance of understanding the anatomy pertinent to CVA placement has never been greater. Comprehending general venous anatomy is important to the practitioner developing a CVA service, but of almost equal importance is being familiar with the wide range of variant anatomy so commonly encountered in the venous system. Additionally, due to the increased incidence of venous thromboses noted in patients who have had prior CVA device placement, collateral pathways that normally would not be used in CVA device placement become increasingly important as possible conduits for catheter placement.

The goal of this chapter is to introduce the reader to the normal anatomy and anatomic relationships of the venous system used in CVA device placement; to discuss commonly occurring anatomic variants; and to introduce collateral pathways important in venous access.

ANTERIOR VENOUS DRAINAGE ABOVE THE DIAPHRAGM

Venous Anatomy of the Neck

The veins of the neck are important pathways for placement of CVA devices. Although they are used for virtually all types of CVA devices, the neck veins are particularly important in placement of hemodialysis catheters because placement of such catheters into the subclavian veins may cause occlusions and preclude placement of future arm grafts or fistulas (3). Placement of CVA devices into the neck are often more easily accomplished than placements in other venous systems due to the superficial location of the neck veins and the relative ease with which the veins can be accessed using either anatomic landmarks or imaging guidance.

The venous system of the neck consists of the *jugular veins.* The jugular system is composed of the internal, external, and anterior jugular veins. Generally speaking, the jugular venous systems are inversely proportioned to one another; if the internal jugular veins are large, the ipsilateral external system tends to be smaller. The *internal jugular vein* (IJV) is formed at the base of the skull as a continuation of the transverse sinus. As the IJV courses caudally, the relationship it shares with the carotid artery typically changes but is completely variable; the IJV may be anterolateral, directly lateral, or posterolateral to the carotid artery anywhere along its course (Fig. 2.1). Between the artery and the vein lies the vagus nerve. Each IJV has one or two valves near its termination, at the confluence of the IJV and subclavian veins. Tributaries

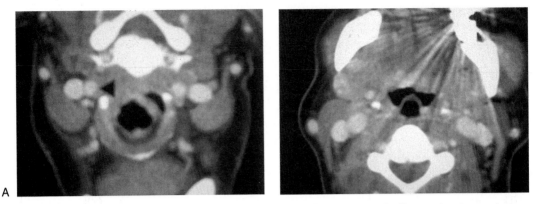

A   B

FIG. 2.1. Relationship of the jugular vein and carotid artery in the neck. Contrast-enhanced computed tomography scan of the neck demonstrates the left internal jugular vein (IJV, *white arrowhead*) to be posterolateral to the carotid artery (*black arrowhead*) in the mid-neck **(A)**, whereas higher in the neck near the skull base the IJV is directly lateral to the carotid artery **(B)**. This relationship is highly variable and changes from patient to patient.

include the inferior petrosal sinus; facial, lingual, and pharyngeal veins; and superior and middle thyroidal veins. On the left, the thoracic duct enters at approximately the level of the confluence of the IJV and subclavian vein; in approximately two thirds of cases the duct drains into the IJV. Although variable, the right IJV tends to be larger in diameter than the left.

The *external jugular vein* (EJV) receives drainage from the scalp and deep veins of the face. It originates at the level of the angle of the mandible, in the substance of the parotid gland. It initially courses along the posterior border of the sternocleidomastoid, but at the level of the mid-neck it crosses the muscle obliquely before entering the deep cervical fascia and ending in the subclavian vein.

The *anterior jugular vein* (AJV) may either be single or paired. It originates near the level of the hyoid bone and lies on or near the midline of the neck. The AJV is variable in size and may even by difficult to visualize. The AJVs, if bilateral, usually form a common trunk in the upper chest before entering the external or subclavian veins. There is a transverse communication between the AJVs termed the *jugular venous arch*, which allows communication between all three jugular systems (Fig. 2.2).

Venous Anatomy of the Upper Extremities

Venous drainage of the upper extremities can be separated into deep and superficial systems. The superficial system consists of the cephalic and basilic systems, whereas the deep system is composed of the brachial veins and the deep venous system of the forearm (Fig. 2.3).

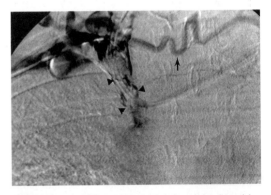

FIG. 2.2. Jugular venous arch, right brachiocephalic vein thrombosis. Digital subtraction venogram through a catheter placed in the central right subclavian vein. There is complete occlusion of the right brachiocephalic vein with thrombus (*arrowheads*), and reconstitution of the left brachiocephalic vein via the jugular venous arch (*arrow*).

The superficial venous system of the upper extremity is frequently used during CVA procedures. This system offers the benefit of being closer to the skin than the corresponding deep venous system; additionally, as opposed to the deep venous system, the superficial system generally does not course adjacent to other vital structures, such as nerves or arteries. In the forearm, the two superficial systems (cephalic and basilic) are frequently connected by anastomoses, the largest of which is the median cubital vein at the level of the elbow.

The *cephalic vein* is formed from the dorsal venous network of the hand and courses along the radial aspect of the wrist and forearm. It continues superficial to the biceps brachii muscle in the upper arm before entering the infraclavicular fossa behind the pectoralis major muscle. It is the major tributary to the axillary vein, entering anywhere from the level of the teres major muscle to the lateral margin of the first rib. Frequently, an *accessory cephalic vein* is noted that arises more laterally than the cephalic vein, draining the dorsolateral aspect of the forearm. The accessory cephalic vein typically joins the cephalic vein above the elbow; however, forearm anastomoses between the two systems are common.

The *basilic vein* is generally the largest single vein of the upper extremity. It forms in the forearm by receiving drainage from the ulnar aspect of the dorsal venous network of the hand. After coursing along the medial aspect of the forearm, it dives deep to lie medial to the biceps brachii muscle. At the level of the midupper arm, the basilic vein pierces the deep fascia and continues medial to the brachial artery and vein. At the level of the inferior border of the teres major muscle, the basilic vein continues as the axillary vein. The median antebrachial cutaneous nerve courses adjacent to the basilic vein.

Unlike the superficial venous system, the deep venous system of the upper extremities is typically accompanied by adjacent nerves and arteries. Because of these relationships, puncture of a vein of the deep venous system is more fraught with risk than puncture of a vein of the superficial system. In the arm, the deep venous system parallels the arterial system. The *deep veins of the forearm* derive their supply from the palmar arches (deep and superficial); the

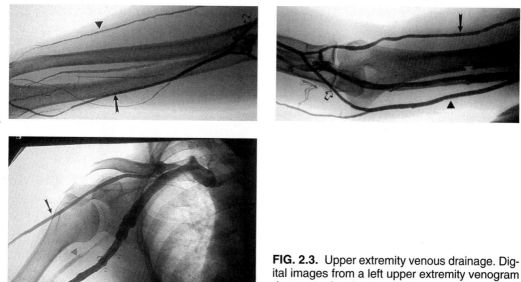

FIG. 2.3. Upper extremity venous drainage. Digital images from a left upper extremity venogram demonstrating the normal venous anatomy of the arm. *Arrow,* cephalic vein; *black arrowhead,* basilic vein; *white arrowhead,* duplicated brachial veins; *open arrow,* median cubital vein.

deep veins are composed of the ulnar vein, typically the largest deep forearm vein, the radial vein, and the anterior and posterior interosseous veins. Similar to the interosseous veins, the radial and ulnar veins are frequently paired. The ulnar vein typically has a branch that joins the median cubital vein, providing a collateral from the deep to superficial systems. The deep veins of the forearm join near the elbow to form the brachial vein.

The *brachial vein* continues above the elbow as the main draining vein of the deep venous system. The brachial vein is often duplicated and therefore is frequently smaller in diameter than the nearby basilic vein. The brachial vein joins the basilic vein around the level of the teres major muscle or the inferior margin of the subscapularis.

As mentioned above, the brachial vein has important anatomic relationships that decrease its desirability as a vein for CVA. In particular, the paired brachial veins normally surround the adjacent brachial artery, making access of one of the veins fairly difficult without endangering the adjacent artery. Additionally, the brachial vein is accompanied by the median nerve. All of these structures (veins, artery, and nerve) are encased by a thick fascial layer in the upper arm termed the medial brachial fascia. This fascial envelope is particularly significant when accessing the brachial veins, because any hematoma arising from puncture of either the vein or artery might be contained within the fascia rather than extending relatively harmlessly into the surrounding soft tissues. Such a hematoma could cause increased pressure within the fascial envelope, leading to arterial compromise or nerve damage. Unlike the brachial vein, the basilic vein is not contained within a fascial compartment, so a hematoma arising from this vein does not necessarily endanger the adjacent cutaneous nerve.

The *axillary vein* is a continuation of the basilic vein at the inferior margin of the teres major muscle. Although the brachial veins usually join the basilic vein at this level, the axillary vein is not by definition formed by the confluence of these venous structures. The axillary vein receives the cephalic vein as its major tributary. The axillary artery lies cephalad and lateral to the vein, and the medial cord of the brachial plexus typically lies between the two vessels.

The axillary vein becomes the subclavian vein at the lateral margin of the first rib.

Venous Anatomy of the Chest

The veins of the thorax receive drainage from the head and neck, upper extremities, and mediastinum. In addition, by receiving flow from the azygous system, the thoracic veins receive drainage from the entire posterior venous system. Because of this connection to the posterior venous system, in cases of inferior vena cava obstruction the thoracic veins receive drainage from literally the entire body.

The *subclavian vein* represents the continuation of the axillary vein, originating at the lateral margin of the first rib and coursing centrally to the junction of the internal jugular vein (Fig. 2.4). The subclavian veins lie largely behind or dorsal to the clavicle, and dorsal and

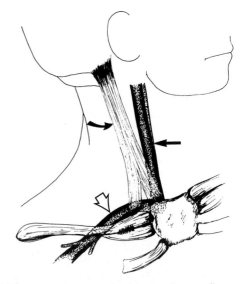

FIG. 2.4. Neck and chest vein confluence. Drawing demonstrating the confluence of the internal jugular vein (*arrow*) and subclavian vein (*open arrow*) at approximately the level of the sternoclavicular junction. *Curved arrow*, sternocleidomastoid muscle.

cephalad to the subclavian artery. The only major tributary to the subclavian vein is the external jugular vein.

At the junction of the subclavian and internal jugular veins, approximately at the level of the sternoclavicular junction, the *brachiocephalic vein* is formed. The right and left brachiocephalic veins, previously called the innominate veins, differ significantly. The right brachiocephalic vein is 2 to 3 cm in length and lies between the sternal head of the clavicle and the anterior margin of the first rib on the right. The left brachiocephalic vein must course across the entire mediastinum before joining its right-sided counterpart. It does so by traversing the mediastinum between the manubrium ventrally and the great arteries of the mediastinum dorsally. The left brachiocephalic vein is approximately 6 cm in length; it joins the right brachiocephalic vein at the level of the right anterior first rib. Major tributaries to the brachiocephalic veins include the vertebral, internal mammary, and inferior thyroidal veins; in addition, the left brachiocephalic vein receives blood from the superior intercostal vein.

The *superior vena cava* (SVC) is formed by the confluence of the right and left brachiocephalic veins. The origin of the SVC is at the level of the first anterior rib on the right. Approximately 7 cm in length, the lower half of the SVC lies within the pericardial space. The SVC does not contain valves. Other than the brachiocephalic veins, the major tributary to the SVC is the azygous vein, which enters at approximately the level of the mid-SVC, just before the latter vein enters the pericardium. Additional small tributaries include branches from the pericardium and mediastinum.

Anomalies of the veins of the chest are largely limited to those involving the SVC. The most common variant involving the SVC is a complete duplication, seen in approximately 0.3% of the population (4). Embryologically, the left-sided SVC develops due to a lack of normal development of the left-sided brachiocephalic vein and persistence of the left anterior cardinal vein. The left-sided SVC drains directly into the coronary sinus. A less common anomaly occurs when the right anterior cardinal vein regresses instead of the left, resulting in an isolated left-sided SVC. As in a duplicated system, the left SVC drains into the coronary sinus.

ANTERIOR VENOUS DRAINAGE BELOW THE DIAPHRAGM

Venous Drainage of the Lower Extremities

Similar to the venous drainage of the upper extremities, drainage of the lower extremities occurs via both a deep and superficial system. Unlike the arms, however, the majority of blood return from the lower extremities occurs via the deep drainage pathway.

The superficial venous system of the lower extremity is composed mainly of the *saphenous vein*. Two distinct saphenous systems exist: the greater (longer) and lesser (shorter) saphenous veins. The lesser saphenous vein originates around the lateral malleolus of the ankle, courses posteriorly, and joins the popliteal vein above the knee joint. The greater saphenous vein originates around the medial malleolus and courses along the entire length of the leg to join the common femoral vein below the inguinal ligament (Fig. 2.5). Valves are numerous throughout both saphenous veins, and multiple communications exist between the two. In addition, multiple perforating veins (venae comitantes) are noted between the saphenous and deep venous systems of the legs.

The deep venous drainage pathways in the leg are rarely if ever used for CVA device placement. The veins parallel the accompanying arteries in the calf (anterior and posterior tibial, peroneal) and are typically duplicated. Below the knee the veins combine to form the popliteal vein. As the popliteal vein courses cephalad, it enters the adductor canal and becomes the superficial femoral vein (named for its accompanying artery). The superficial femoral vein continues along the medial aspect of the thigh until it is joined by the greater saphenous vein to become the common femoral vein, just below the inguinal ligament. Other than the saphenous vein, the femoral vein receives many muscular branch tributaries as well as the deep (profunda) femoral vein.

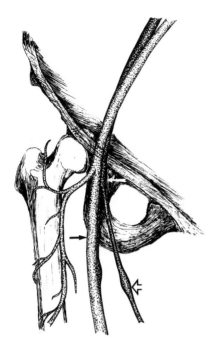

FIG. 2.5. Venous anatomy at the groin. Drawing demonstrating the relationship of the femoral artery (*arrow*) and femoral vein (*white arrow*). Notice how the femoral artery is lateral and partially overlies the femoral vein at the level of the inguinal ligament. *Open arrow,* greater saphenous vein.

The *iliac venous system* begins as the extension of the common femoral vein at the inguinal ligament. The iliac venous system is named according to the adjacent arterial structures, and consists of the external, internal, and common iliac veins. Valves may be found in the external iliac veins, but none are noted in the common iliac veins. The right iliac venous system courses almost vertically out of the pelvis, but the left-sided system has a more oblique orientation. Also of importance, the right common iliac artery crosses the left common iliac vein at the level of the pelvic inlet. Because of this relationship, symptomatic compression of the left common iliac vein may be caused by the overlying artery (May-Thurner syndrome) (5).

The inferior vena cava (IVC) is formed by the confluence of the common iliac veins. This confluence is usually noted at about the level of

the fifth lumbar vertebral body. The IVC is a very capacious vein that can change diameter depending on the cardiac cycle or respiratory variations. The IVC is retroperitoneal throughout its course in the abdomen before entering the substance of the liver. It lies dorsal to the duodenum, pancreas, and lesser sac. Upon entering the liver, the IVC courses in a groove posterior to the caudate lobe. During its intrahepatic course, the IVC angles ventrally and medially to exit the liver and enter the pericardium. The IVC is without valves except for the rudimentary semilunar valve, which lies at the junction of the IVC and right atrium. Because of its dorsal location, there is nothing between the infrarenal IVC and the skin surface of the flank other than pararenal fat and paraspinous musculature. This paucity of important adjacent structures makes direct puncture of the IVC a safe alternative pathway for placement of CVA devices (see Chapter 12).

The *hepatic veins* are sometimes used for venous access in the absence of other available access routes (6). The hepatic veins receive drainage from both the hepatic arterial and portal venous systems, returning blood to the systemic circulation. The hepatic veins lie in the anatomic planes between the hepatic segments, so their drainage distributions do not follow the hepatic arterial distributions. The caudate lobe has a separate drainage pattern, with many small perforating veins draining directly into the IVC rather than forming a separate draining vein. There are typically three hepatic veins: right, middle, and left. Although variations are the norm, the most common drainage pattern is for the right hepatic vein to drain directly into the IVC, while the left and middle hepatic veins combine before entering the IVC (Fig. 2.6). Finally, there can be an accessory (superior) right hepatic vein that drains the most cephalad portion of the liver.

Variant anatomy of the venous system below the diaphragm is relatively rare. In order to best understand such venous anomalies, a brief review of development of the normal venous system is required. The retroperitoneal veins develop from four sets of paired veins, all of which develop at different times of embryo-

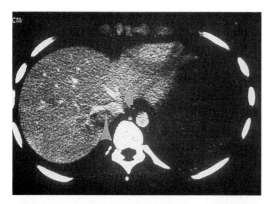

FIG. 2.6. Hepatic vein anatomy. Contrast-enhanced computed tomography scan, filmed at liver window, demonstrates the typical confluence of the left and middle hepatic veins (*arrow*) before entering the inferior vena cava. *Arrowhead,* right hepatic vein.

logic development. The first to form are the *posterior cardinal veins*, which drain the caudal portion of the developing embryo. These paired veins form by the fourth week of development but eventually regress entirely. The *subcardinal veins* develop about the fifth week and drain the same distribution as the earlier posterior cardinal veins; the subcardinal vein on the right eventually forms the middle part of the retroperitoneal IVC, as well as the renal veins. The *sacrocardinal veins* develop about the same time as the subcardinal veins; the sacrocardinal veins drain the lower extremities, pelvis, and develop into the infrarenal portion of the IVC. Finally, the *supracardinal veins,* which develop concurrent with the posterior cardinal veins by 4 weeks, evolve into the azygous/hemiazygous systems. Connections between the right and left cardinal systems, as well as regressions of certain veins during development, are predictable and account for the largely right-sided subdiaphragmatic venous drainage.

The most common anomalies involving the subdiaphragmatic veins occur because of lack of regression of veins during normal development. The most common anomaly is a *duplicated IVC*, which occurs due to a persistence of the left sacrocardinal vein. In a duplicated system, the left sacrocardinal vein maintains it's

connection with the left subcardinal vein; the latter vein eventually forms the left renal vein, accounting for the adult pattern of drainage of a left-sided IVC into the left renal vein. A less common anomaly is an isolated *left-sided IVC,* in which the right-sided subcardinal and sacrocardinal veins regress completely. The final relatively common anomaly is absence of the intrahepatic portion of the IVC, also called *interrupted IVC with azygous continuation.* In this setting, the right subcardinal vein fails to form communication with the developing intrahepatic veins. The drainage from the subhepatic veins is therefore shunted to the supracardinal system, which eventually develops into the azygous system. Drainage of the entire subdiaphragmatic venous system, therefore, is via the azygous system.

POSTERIOR VENOUS DRAINAGE

The venous drainage of the dorsal aspect of the pelvis, abdomen, and chest is via the *azygous venous system.* The azygous system includes the azygous, hemiazygous, and accessory hemiazygous veins. These veins have many interconnections and form a rich network of vessels adjacent to the vertebral column.

The largest of the three veins is the *azygous vein.* The azygous vein lies on the right side of the vertebral column, and is formed by the right ascending lumbar vein at approximately the level of the first or second lumbar vertebra. The azygous vein continues in a cephalad direction, entering the thorax through the aortic hiatus of the diaphragm. At approximately the level of the fourth thoracic vertebra, the azygous vein courses anteriorly (ventrally) to enter the superior vena cava cephalad to the pericardium. The azygous vein receives venous drainage from the right lumbar and intercostal veins, as well as the highest superior intercostal vein on the right (formed by the first through third intercostal veins). The azygous vein also receives blood from several mediastinal veins. The largest tributary to the azygous vein is the hemiazygous vein, which enters at approximately the level of the ninth or tenth thoracic vertebra.

The *hemiazygous vein* begins as an extension of the left ascending lumbar vein. Similar to the left sided azygous vein, the hemiazygous vein receives blood from the left intercostal veins, the upper lumbar veins, and some mediastinal branches. After entering the thoracic cavity via the left crus of the diaphragm, in the lower thoracic region the hemiazygous vein crosses the midline to join the azygous vein.

Cephalad to where the hemiazygous vein crosses the midline, the *accessory hemiazygous vein* descends along the left margin of the vertebral column. The accessory hemiazygous vein receives tributaries from the upper left intercostal veins, as well as some small mediastinal branches. It terminates either in the hemiazygous vein before the latter vein crosses the midline, or the accessory hemiazygous vein crosses the midline and drains directly into the azygous vein. The accessory hemiazygous vein is extremely variable in size, and may even be completely absent. There is an inverse relationship with the size of the accessory hemiazygous and the left highest intercostal vein, depending on the drainage patterns.

COLLATERAL VENOUS DRAINAGE PATTERNS

In the setting of venous obstruction, collateral pathways develop in fairly predictable patterns. This is particularly important during placement of CVA devices; not only may obstructed or stenotic veins become obstacles to device placement, but previous central venous catheter placement is perhaps the most common predisposing factor for central venous occlusion (7–9). Recognizing collateral drainage patterns is important during CVA device placement, because often large collateral pathways may prove to be appropriate for device placement.

Superior vena cava, brachiocephalic, and subclavian vein occlusions account for the vast majority of central catheter-related venous obstructions. When considering *superior vena cava obstructions,* it is important to consider where in the course of the SVC the obstruction occurs. If the blockage is between the azygous conflu-

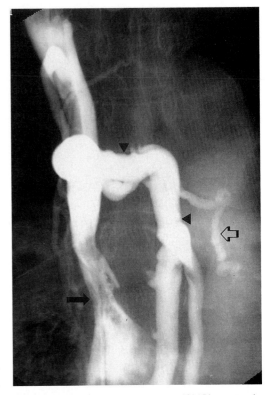

FIG. 2.7. Superior vena cava (SVC) stenosis with retrograde flow through the azygous vein. Unsubtracted digital venogram demonstrating severe distal SVC stenosis (*arrow*) in a patient with long-term central venous access for hemodialysis. Note the extensive posterior collateral formation by the hemiazygous system (*arrowheads*). The enlarged vein draining into the hemiazygous system (*open arrow*) represents either an enlarged bronchial or mediastinal vein. (Courtesy of Charles Owens, M.D.)

ence and the right atrium, flow from the brachiocephalic veins can enter the azygous vein and proceed in retrograde fashion down the posterior system, eventually reaching the IVC via the posterior body wall or retroperitoneal collateral pathways (Fig. 2.7). Conversely, if SVC flow is obstructed cephalad to the azygous confluence, blood must bypass the obstruction via collaterals that form on the chest wall; these chest wall collaterals anastomose with abdominal wall veins, eventually draining into the IVC or azygous system below the diaphragm (Fig. 2.8). In addition, with an SVC ob-

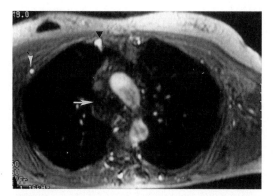

FIG. 2.8. Superior vena cava (SVC) obstruction with chest wall collateral veins. Breath hold gradient echo magnetic resonance image demonstrating SVC obstruction (*arrow*) with collateral flow via the internal mammary vein (*black arrowhead*) and lateral thoracic vein (*white arrowhead*). (Courtesy of Joshua Farber, M.D.)

struction cephalad to the azygous confluence, flow may reverse in the left superior intercostal veins to drain into the accessory hemiazygous vein.

Brachiocephalic vein obstruction typically causes reversal of flow in the jugular venous system. In the setting of unilateral flow, collateral veins typically develop from one jugular system to the other. This cross-filling of jugular systems is most commonly seen as filling of the contralateral external or anterior jugular vein via the jugular venous arch, an anterior vein that courses anterior and inferior to the thyroid. In addition, extensive collateral vessels may form through the thyroidal veins; the superior and middle thyroid veins typically drain into the ipsilateral internal jugular, and the paired inferior thyroid veins may drain separately or into a common trunk before draining into the

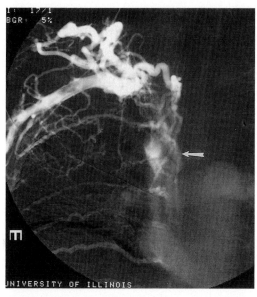

FIG. 2.9. Right brachiocephalic vein obstruction with posterior collateral development. Digital subtraction venography demonstrating right brachiocephalic vein occlusion. Note the extensive posterior chest wall collateral drainage via the intercostal veins with reconstitution of the azygous system (*arrow*). (Courtesy of Charles Owens, M.D.)

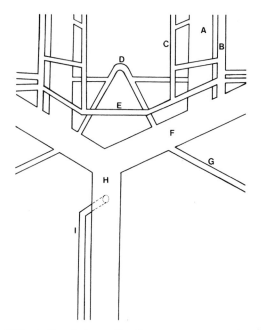

FIG. 2.10. Schematic diagram demonstrating the venous drainage pathways of the upper extremities and neck. Note in particular the extensive interconnections between the various venous drainage systems. **A:** Internal jugular vein. **B:** External jugular vein. **C:** Anterior jugular vein. **D:** Jugular venous arch. **E:** Thyroidal veins. **F:** Brachiocephalic vein. **G:** Internal mammary vein. **H:** Superior vena cava. **I:** Azygous vein.

brachiocephalic veins. Finally, posterior collateral pathways may develop that drain into the azygous system (Fig. 2.9).

Subclavian vein obstruction is likely the most common level for central venous obstruction following catheter placement. The most common collateral networks to develop following subclavian vein obstruction are to the ipsilateral jugular system, typically via neck collateral veins from the thyrocervical trunk. A large collateral vein also may form from the cephalic vein to the jugular system; this unnamed vein may become rather large and may mimic the subclavian vein on magnetic resonance imaging (MRI) or ultrasonography (US). Finally, chest wall collateral veins may form from the axillary vein via lateral thoracic or thoracodorsal tributaries, with drainage via the azygous system or IVC tributaries.

Figure 2.10 represents a schematic diagram of venous connections, and therefore potential collateral pathways, of veins above the diaphragm.

ACKNOWLEDGMENT

I thank Stacy Erickson for the medical illustrations accompanying the text.

REFERENCES

1. Kalso E. A short history of central venous catheterization. *Acta Anesthesiol Scand* 1985;81(suppl):7–10.
2. Hickman RO, Buckner ED, Clift RA, et al. A modified right atrial catheter for access to the venous system in marrow transplant recipients. *Surg Gynecol Obstet* 1979;148:871–875.
3. Trerotola SO, Johnson MS, Harris VJ, et al. Outcome of tunneled hemodialysis catheters placed via the right internal jugular vein by interventional radiologists. *Radiology* 1997;203:489–495.
4. Kadir S. *Atlas of normal and variant angiographic anatomy.* Philadelphia: WB Saunders, 1991:163.
5. Ferris EJ, Lim WN, Smith PL, et al. May-Thurner syndrome. *Radiology* 1983;147:29–31.
6. Kaufman JA, Greenfield AJ, Fitzpatrick GF. Transhepatic cannulation of the inferior vena cava. *J Vasc Intervent Radiol* 1991;2:331–334.
7. Lyon RD, Griggs KA, Johnson AM, et al. Long-term follow-up of upper extremity implanted venous access devices in oncology patients. *J Vasc Intervent Radiol* 1999;10:463–471.
8. Lokich JJ, Bothe A Jr, Benotti P, et al. Complications and management of implanted venous access catheters. *J Clin Oncol* 1985;3:710–717.
9. McLean Ross AH, Griffith CDM, et al. Thromboembolic complications with silicone elastomer subclavian catheters. *J Parenter Enter Nutr* 1982;6:61–63.

SUGGESTED READINGS

Kadir S. *Diagnostic angiography.* Philadelphia: WB Saunders, 1986.
Kadir S. *Atlas of normal and variant angiographic anatomy.* Philadelphia: WB Saunders, 1991.
Pick TP, Howden R. *Grays anatomy, descriptive and surgical,* 15th ed. New York: Bounty Books, 1977.
Sadler TW. *Langman's medical embryology,* 5th ed. Baltimore: Williams & Wilkins, 1985:203–209.

Central Venous Access
Edited by Charles E. Ray, Jr.
Lippincott Williams & Wilkins, Philadelphia © 2001.

3

Imaging Guidance
for Central Venous Access

Thomas B. Kinney, MD

Department of Vascular and Interventional Radiology, UCSD Medical Center,
San Diego, California 92103

Single-lumen central venous catheters were introduced in the 1970s. The development of dual-lumen, tunneled, cuffed catheters followed in the 1980s. The availability of these central venous catheters is crucial in the management of a wide variety of clinical situations. Central lines are used for intravenous (IV) medications such as chemotherapeutic agents, antibiotics, blood products, and total parenteral nutrition; IV therapies such as hemodialysis or pheresis; and for frequent blood sampling. The availability of these permanent central catheters simplifies the care of patients who can receive medical therapies outside the acute care facility, greatly reducing costs. In the past two decades, the use of long-term venous access devices has increased dramatically. Whereas more than 5 million central venous catheters are sold in the United States annually (1), it has been estimated that approximately 500,000 long-term venous access catheters are inserted each year (2). The use of such devices continues to grow annually, a trend that is readily apparent to physicians providing venous access service. It is expected that the use of such devices will continue to grow given patient demographics and the evolution of newer IV therapies.

Traditionally, central venous catheters were placed by surgeons in operating rooms. Access into the venous system was performed either by direct cut-down or by percutaneous technique using landmarks rather than imaging guidance. Final catheter position was confirmed with flu-oroscopy or spot films. In this era, radiologic methods were used infrequently for problem solving. This included outlining venous anatomy by contrast venography either before or after failed central venous access (CVA), catheter fragment retrieval, and redirection of misplaced catheters.

Currently, the radiologist's role in CVA has expanded because of a multiplicity of factors. Familiarity with the Seldinger technique (3) and venous anatomy in conjunction with advances in imaging such as sonography and fluoroscopy has allowed radiologists to insert such devices more efficaciously and with similar or lower complication rates than surgically placed lines. CVA obtained within the radiologic suite can often be performed quicker than in a busy operating room, and the access can frequently be performed the day the request is made. Moreover, the use of the interventional suite may result in savings because the costs of both the operating room and the anesthesiologist are not incurred (4).

The goals of this chapter are to describe imaging guidance for CVA. The utility of imaging becomes apparent even before the procedure is undertaken. Review of imaging studies supplemented by additional studies in select cases facilitate planning the procedure. Next, the methods of image directed venous access are presented and compared with landmark based methods. The use of imaging to facilitate accurate catheter placement once access has been obtained are then discussed. After completing this chapter, the reader should be comfortable planning, performing, and documenting CVA procedures.

PREPROCEDURAL REVIEW

Several factors aid in the decision as to which sites should be considered for creation of the access (Table 3.1). Many of the important factors can be elicited by history and physical examination findings. For example, a patient with a history of multiple previous lines may have a reduced number of possible access sites secondary to prior catheter-related thrombosis. Significant clinical details also include prior surgery or radiation therapy of the head, neck, or chest. Patients with malignant mediastinal tumors (lymphoma), head and neck tumors, or apical lung tumors also may have limited access sites because of tumor encasement or extrinsic compression of the central veins. A prior history of upper extremity edema with or without head and neck swelling may indicate prior central conduit vein thrombosis. Several reasons exist why accesses should not be placed ipsilateral to planned or prior breast surgery. Lymphedema occurs in up to 60% of women who have undergone radical mastectomy and up to 30% of women who have been treated with modified radical mastectomy or breast-conserving surgery (5). The lymphedema may be exacerbated by venous access created ipsilateral to mastectomy. Furthermore, the risk of infection increases with the presence of lymph-edema. The access device also can potentially interfere with planned radiation portals. Most importantly, the patient's preference must be considered because patient satisfaction with the access site is crucial (6).

Physical examination findings may help select the optimal access site. The presence of cutaneous pathology (primary or metastatic tumors), graft-versus-host disease, burns, plastic surgery skin flaps, tattoos, cellulitis, etc. may eliminate certain sites. The presence of upper extremity edema or visible, dilated collateral veins in the shoulder, chest, or neck may indicate central venous occlusion. The examination also includes visual inspection of the anticipated tunnel sites. A detailed explanation of the planned sites is important to the patient because certain life-style issues may come into play. For instance, a chest port on the side of a patient who uses recreational firearms may cause complications and constant irritation to the patient. Similarly, visible subcutaneously tunneled catheters or scars in patients who desire to wear low-cut blouses may be aggravating to patients, serving as constant reminders of their disease condition or eliciting embarrassing questions from friends or family members.

Review of the patient's radiography file may indicate prior CVA sites not recalled by the patient. These are easily detected by reviewing chest radiographs, which also may reveal important mediastinal or chest pathology. Hemodialysis patients frequently have venograms performed during dialysis graft declotting and maintenance, and review of these may indicate whether certain access conduits are patent. Many oncology patients will have undergone chest computed tomography (CT) studies, which may reveal chest or mediastinal pathology important for planning the access.

In patients with clinically suspected or evident central venous thrombosis, additional imaging workup may be necessary to plan for successful CVA. Although contrast venography has traditionally been used to establish the diagnosis of central venous thrombosis, ultrasonography (US) is the imaging procedure of choice presently in the workup of such cases (7).

TABLE 3.1. *Important considerations for pre-procedure planning for CVA*

Historical features
    Previous central venous catheters
    Previous surgery or radiation therapy of the head, neck, or chest
    Known venous anomalies
    Mediastinal, neck, or chest pathology
    Prior mastectomy
    History of upper extremity, head, or neck swelling
Physical examination findings
    Primary or metastatic cutaneous disease
    Burns
    Upper extremity edema
    Dilated shoulder, chest, or neck venous collaterals
Patient preference

IMAGING METHODS TO EVALUATE FOR SUSPECTED CENTRAL VENOUS PROBLEMS

Ultrasonography

Familiarity with US techniques for assessing the upper extremity veins is imperative to the success of the interventional radiologist performing CVA. The technique is best accomplished with high-resolution US equipment such as phased-array transducers using frequencies of 7.5 MHz or higher for gray-scale imaging (8). A small footprint for the transducer facilitates imaging vessels beneath the clavicle and sternum. Lower frequency probes may be necessary in larger patients. A 10- or 7.5-MHz linear-array probe can be used to examine the internal jugular veins (IJVs) and usually the lateral segments of the subclavian veins.

The typical US examination includes the IJVs, brachiocephalic veins (BCVs), subclavian veins, and axillary veins. Both sides are studied because subtle asymmetry in the Doppler spectra may indicate more central thrombosis or stenosis that may not be directly visualized. The sternum and clavicles may make direct visualization of the superior vena cava (SVC), BCVs, and medial portions of the subclavian veins difficult or impossible.

The three components of a US examination of the upper extremity veins are the real-time observation of the veins with gray-scale imaging, the color Doppler imaging, and the Doppler waveform analysis. Normal subclavian veins and IJVs have hypoechoic lumina and have valves that open and close completely. Doppler sonography permits evaluation of reflected right atrium (RA) waveforms and flow changes associated with respiration (Fig. 3.1). The RA waveforms reflect changing pressures within the RA and are called a, c, and v atrial pressure waves. The a wave is caused by RA contraction. The c wave occurs when the ventricles begin to contract. These are felt to be caused by the bulging back of the tricuspid valve because of the increasing pressure in the ventricle and the pulling on the atrial muscles by the contracting right ventricle. The v wave occurs toward the end of ventricular contraction

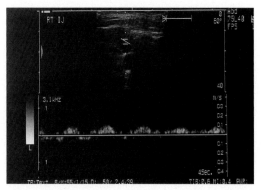

FIG. 3.1. Transverse US view of the right internal jugular vein, which is interrogated with Doppler. The waveform shows atrial phasicity and subtle respiratory variation consistent with a widely patent conduit to the central venous circulation. The flow rate is a maximum of 100 cm/s, with 6 atrial beats in 34 seconds (heart rate of 90 beats/min) and respiratory variation of 1 in 4 seconds (15 respirations/min).

and results from the slow buildup of blood within the RA while the tricuspid valve is closed during ventricular contraction. The buildup of pressure with each a, c, and v wave reduces flow toward the RA. The process of inspiration reduces intrathoracic pressure, augmenting flow toward the RA. The atria contract at an average rate of 1 Hz (60 beats/min, with three atrial waveforms with each beat), whereas the respiratory variation is much slower at an average of 0.2 Hz (12 breaths/ min). The diameter of the subclavian vein normally changes with respiration and in response to the Valsalva maneuver, forced expiration, and sniffing (9). A normal subclavian vein decreases an average of 61% (range 41%–78%) in caliber during sniffing. This is reported to be the most reliable real-time measurement for assessing vein patency, but this maneuver may be limited in certain patients. A mean increase in diameter of 21% (range -5% to +43.5%) is seen with the Valsalva maneuver. Color Doppler aids in rapid localization of the vessels, in differentiation of arteries from veins, and in delineation of thrombus.

The patient is examined in the supine position without elevation of the head, which is rotated away from the side of examination. The

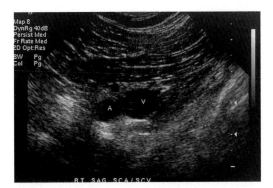

FIG. 3.2. Sagittal view of the right subclavian vein and artery shows that the artery is normally smaller, deeper, and more cephalad than the acompanying subclavian vein, which is larger, more superficial, and more caudal.

IJV is very superficial, and is easily visualized and compressed by the transducer. The IJV is located by scanning transversely and is evaluated by compression cephalad to caudad to exclude occlusive or nonocclusive thrombus (10). The vessel is interrogated with Doppler imaging in the longitudinal plane without inducing any venous compression by the probe over the vein. The BCV is next examined, and a Doppler signature obtained both from a medial acoustic window (suprasternal) with the probe angled inferiorly on the right side and inferiorly and medially on the left side. The ipsilateral subclavian vein is located at its junction with the IJV, with the probe placed transversely and just medial to the clavicular head. Depending on body habitus, the BCVs may or may not be seen. The remainder of the subclavian vein is examined from a lateral infraclavicular window. Doppler signals are recorded from the middle and lateral segments of the subclavian veins. The normal anatomic relationship of the subclavian vein to the subclavian artery must be understood (Fig. 3.2). The subclavian artery is more cephalad, deeper (posterior), and smaller in caliber than the accompanying vein. The faster pulsations of the artery can be appreciated and contrasted to the slower respiratory changes in the caliber of the vein. Large venous collaterals may arise in patients with prior subclavian vein thrombosis, and these vessels will be of smaller size and in atypical locations

relative to the artery. The axillary vein typically is less pulsatile than the subclavian vein.

Gray-scale US signs of thrombosis include variable echogenic intraluminal thrombus, absence of beating valves, noncompressibility, absence of response to the Valsalva or sniff maneuvers, and loss of respiratory variability and vessel pulsation (Fig. 3.3). With acute or chronic thrombosis, the high-contrast interface between the venous lumen and the posterior venous wall disappears abruptly (cutoff sign) (11). In cases involving chronic occlusions, collateral vessels may be found and the thrombosed vessel may not be visualized. Veins located peripherally to central venous obstructions may appear dilated and stand out as potential candidates for the unwary interventionalist to access. Careful examination for abnormal response to respiratory maneuvers or absence of transmitted atrial pulsations may reveal the presence of central obstruction not directly visualized (Fig. 3.4). Total venous obstruction results in absence of flow, and partial occlusion of a long segment results in abnormal Doppler waveforms peripheral to the occluded segments that do not vary with respiration and lack atrial pulsations. Occasionally, a stenosis is detected by increased flow velocity and turbulence (Fig. 3.5). Symmetrically damped waveforms detected bilaterally in the IJVs, brachial veins, and subclavian veins may indicate compression or stenosis of the SVC, although the sensitivity and specificity of Doppler sonography for SVC stenoses has not yet been described. False-positive results are rare with Doppler US. False-negative results may occur in patients with small nonobstructive clots or in patients with extensive collateral networks. In cases where US does not adequately delineate a possible site for CVA, additional workup with contrast venography, CT, or magnetic resonance imaging (MRI) may be required.

Conventional Contrast Venography

Contrast venography of the upper extremities is generally used after nondiagnostic US studies in patients with swollen upper extremities (Fig. 3.5) (12). Additional goals may be to map

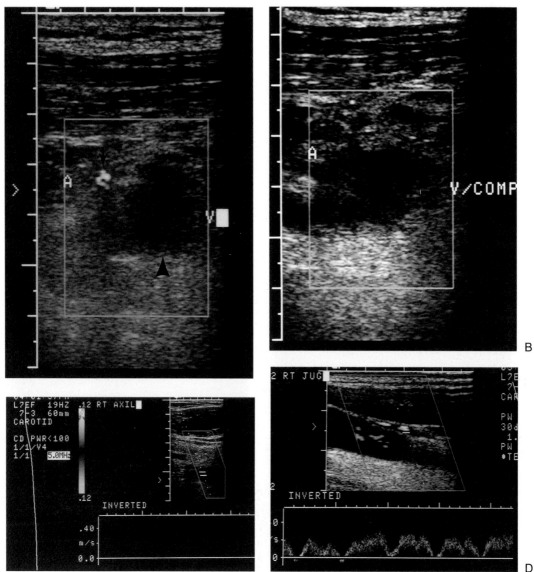

FIG. 3.3. A: Sagittal view of the right subclavian vein in a 44-year-old man with a swollen right upper extremity. The vein (*arrowhead*) is dilated when compared with the artery (*arrow*). The clot is this case is hypoechoic. **B:** Sagittal view of the right subclavian vein during a compression maneuver shows lack of normal compressibility. **C:** Gated Doppler examination of the right axillary vein shows no flow. **D:** The right internal jugular vein is patent with a normal atrial phasicity (4 beats in 4 seconds or a heart rate of 60 beats/min).

out the venous system for planning venous access for fistulas or arteriovenous bypass grafts. Lastly, patients with clinical evidence for SVC syndrome may be studied with contrast venography (13, 14). The symptoms that lead one to suspect SVC syndrome include cyanosis and swelling of the head, neck, and upper extremities, along with the appearance of multiple dilated superficial venous collaterals near the junction of the neck and chest.

If the veins of the forearm need to be studied, an IV in the distal forearm is chosen. For evaluation of the axillary vein or more central venous structures, the cubitak or proximal forearm veins may be used. In general, the IV should be at least 19 gauge to achieve the flow rates required to visualize the central veins upon contrast injection. With the arm in a neutral palmer position, contrast hand injections with digital acquisition with or without tourniquets is performed. The tourniquets may aid in filling the deeper venous structures (brachial vein and axillary vein) because the upper extremity is predominantly drained by the superficial venous conduits (basilic and cephalic veins). In general, nonionic contrast is used [Omnipaque 320 (Mallinkrodt Inc., St. Louis, MO, U.S.A.) can be diluted], but ionic contrast also can be used (Conray 43, Mallinkrodt). To facilitate visualization of the subclavian vein, the arm can be elevated approximately 30 degrees to ease drainage. The arm is usually abducted 90 degrees with respect to the thorax when these studies are performed. Manual compression of the contrast-filled forearm or upper arm also may help to fill the central veins. The SVC can be evaluated by simultaneous bilateral cubital vein injections. An alternative technique involves simultaneous injections of contrast media into basilic veins, cephalic veins, or

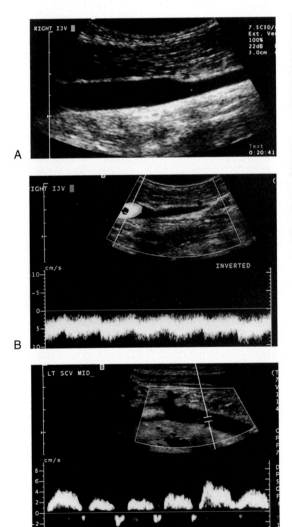

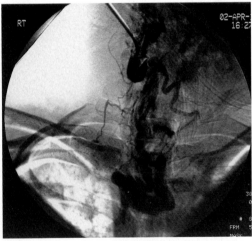

FIG. 3.4. Twenty-four-year-old hemodialysis patient with a failed peripheral access site who required hemodialysis catheter insertion. **A:** The proximal right internal jugular vein (IJV) shown in a longitudinal projection is dilated, appearing as a good potential candidate for access. The left IJV was occluded (not shown). **B:** The Doppler examination demonstrates a dampened waveform (monophasic, with no reversal of flow), which suggests poor venous outflow. **C:** The Doppler waveform from the right subclavian vein is shown for comparison (triphasic, with reversal of flow). **D:** Venogram after failed attempted right IJV catheter placement documents the suspected central venous occlusion.

brachial veins using 4 to 5 French (Fr) straight catheters with or without multiple sideholes.

In patients who are unable to receive iodinated contrast material because of allergic reactions or renal failure, contrast agents such as carbon dioxide (15) or gadolinium (Mallinkrodt) (16) can be used to perform venograms (Fig. 3.6).

Contrast Computed Tomography

Contrast-enhanced CT in an alternative method to contrast venography and US to assess the patency of central veins. CT may provide useful information on vessel patency, vessel size, and collateral pathways (Fig. 3.7). Advantages of CT over US include the ability to see beyond bone and air. CT has some limitations because of the need for iodinated contrast material, as well as artifacts (streak artifact and flow-related artifacts) that occur during contrast injections (17,18).

Magnetic Resonance Imaging Venography

Several groups have investigated the use of MRI for delineation of the central venous structures (Fig. 3.8) (19–24). MRI is not limited in patients with contrast allergies or renal insuffi-

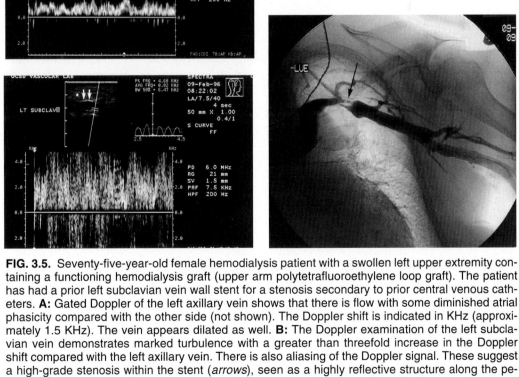

FIG. 3.5. Seventy-five-year-old female hemodialysis patient with a swollen left upper extremity containing a functioning hemodialysis graft (upper arm polytetrafluoroethylene loop graft). The patient has had a prior left subclavian vein wall stent for a stenosis secondary to prior central venous catheters. **A:** Gated Doppler of the left axillary vein shows that there is flow with some diminished atrial phasicity compared with the other side (not shown). The Doppler shift is indicated in KHz (approximately 1.5 KHz). The vein appears dilated as well. **B:** The Doppler examination of the left subclavian vein demonstrates marked turbulence with a greater than threefold increase in the Doppler shift compared with the left axillary vein. There is also aliasing of the Doppler signal. These suggest a high-grade stenosis within the stent (*arrows*), seen as a highly reflective structure along the peripheral vein surface. **C:** The subclavian vein venogram demonstrates a high-grade lesion presumed to be secondary to intimal hyperplasia within the subclavian vein wall stent (*arrow*). The lesion responded well to balloon angioplasty.

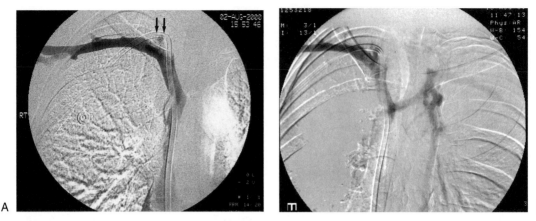

FIG. 3.6. An example of a gadolinium right arm venogram. The patient is a 39-year-old woman with chronic Guillain-Barré syndrome treated with pheresis therapy. She had symptoms of intermittent SVC syndrome and was also allergic to iodinated contrast (prior reaction complicated by laryngeal edema). **A:** The examination shows mild narrowing of the right brachiocephalic vein and SVC. A right internal jugular vein pheresis catheter is in place (*arrows*). **B:** The patient returned 16 days later with recurrent symptoms of SVC syndrome, and repeat gadolinium venography at this time showed occlusion of the SVC with filling of mediastinal venous collaterals that fill the hemiazygous vein. The patient responded well to balloon angioplasty.

ciency, although not all patients can be placed in the MRI scanner because of pacemakers, metallic foreign bodies, or claustrophobias. The most frequently reported method has used a two-dimensional time of flight (2-D TOF) sequence, which is a flow-sensitive method that does not require IV contrast. This is an added benefit in these patients, where venous access is the predominant problem eliciting the referral. In general, the studies thus far reported, which all consist of relatively small series of patients, have reported excellent correlation between the results obtained with MRI and conventional contrast venography. Moreover, the studies readily demonstrate an impact on the planned access procedure. In most cases, the coronal, axial, and sagittal planes are imaged and presaturation bands must be applied adjacent to the imaged slices to suppress adjacent arterial signals. Finn reported on 30 patients suspected of having thoracic venous pathology and corroborated 86% of the cases with a 2-D TOF venographic study (20). Hartnell et al. reported a 100% agreement between 2-D TOF MRI and contrast venograms in all 17 cases where veno-

graphic correlation was available (22). Rose used a 2-D TOF technique and demonstrated a 97% sensitivity and 94% specificity for detection of occlusions (21). However, a high rate of interobserver variability (44%) was reported because of complex drainage patterns in such patients with obstructed central veins.

More recently, Lebowitz described a faster method using a dynamic gadolinium-enhanced three-dimensional gradient echo MRI with subtraction of the arterial phase images to obtain gadolinium-enhanced venograms (24). This method can potentially provide comprehensive imaging of the central veins within a few breath holds.

TRADITIONAL METHODS OF CENTRAL VENOUS ACCESS

Historically, access into the central veins including subclavian veins and IJVs has been performed without imaging guidance using anatomic references. The anatomy of these sites is reviewed in Chapter 1. Access into either of these venous sites can be obtained either by

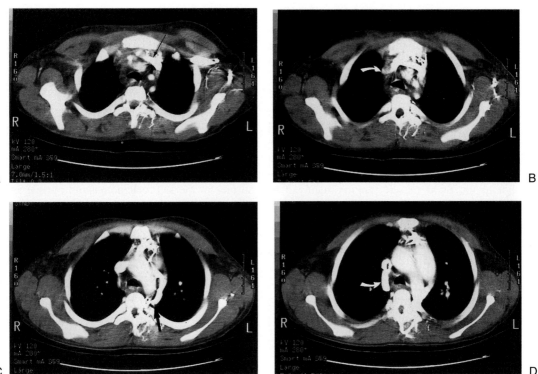

FIG. 3.7. An example of a contrast computed tomogram to evaluate for central venous access (same patient as shown in Fig. 3.4). The left upper extremity is being injected. **A:** At the base of the neck, the left brachiocephalic vein (BCV) (*arrow*) fills with contrast, whereas the right internal jugular vein (IJV) is not seen. **B:** The junction of the left BCV and the SVC (*arrow*) fills. The right IJV is occluded. **C:** The SVC is patent, and the patient has a large left supreme intercostal vein collateral that fills the left hemiazygous system (*arrow*). **D:** The patient also has a large azygous vein (*arrow*) that drains into the SVC, acting as a major collateral pathway to drain the upper extremities. Based on these findings, an inferior vena cava hemodialysis catheter was inserted and a left upper extremity hemodialysis graft was planned.

cutdown onto the vein or with the Seldinger method (3).

Internal Jugular Vein Cannulation

Either IJV is suitable for temporary or permanent venous access, although the right IJV is preferred because its course to the SVC and RA is short and straight (25).

Percutaneous puncture of the IJV can be obtained by directing a needle at the apex of the triangle of the angle made by the sternal and clavicular heads of the sternocleidomastoid (SCM) muscle. This method is referred to as the medial approach. The needle is directed toward the ipsilateral nipple and advanced at a 45 de-

gree angle to the body surface until the vein is entered. The ability to place the patient in the Trendelenburg position at the time of puncture may facilitate the technique by distending the vein maximally (26). In general, the IJV is lateral to the common carotid artery (CCA), but variations do occur. Alternatively, a vertical incision can be made just above the clavicle between the sternal and clavicular heads of the SCM muscle for direct IJV cutdown. The platysma is divided and the CCA sheath carefully located and divided longitudinally, exposing the IJV. The vagus nerve typically lies posteromedial to the IJV, although variation occurs, and this nerve is carefully dissected free from the IJV. Vessel loops are used to secure proximal and distal control of the IJV and a purse-string proline suture is placed with adequate room left within the purse-string to insert a catheter. The catheter is inserted after tunneling and the purse-string tightened to obtain hemostasis.

Alternative percutaneous approaches to the IJV include both the posterior and anterior approaches. The posterior approach is performed by cannulation of the IJV from the posterior border of the SCM muscle at the level of the thyroid cartilage. The needle is directed posterior to the SCM muscle, approximately 3 to 4 cm above the clavicle with the needle directed toward the suprasternal notch until blood return is noted from the needle. With the anterior approach, the IJV is cannulated at the anterior

border of the sternocleidomastoid muscle with the neck in an extended but neutral position. The CCA needs to be palpated and displaced medially to prevent inadvertent CCA puncture. The needle is advanced toward the ipsilateral nipple from a point midway on a line traced from the angle of the mandible to the clavicle.

The external jugular vein (EJV) can often be located visually in the upper, lateral neck. Cannulation of this vein provides access to the central conduit veins because this vein follows the surface of the sternocleidomastoid muscle and flows parallel to the IJV, both of which empty into the neck. The EJV can be cannulated directly at any point along its course, where it is readily apparent visually.

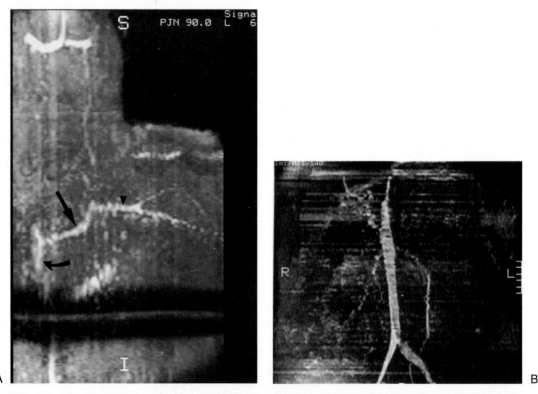

A   B

FIG. 3.8. The patient is a 52-year-old man with chronic renal insufficiency who had a failed left upper arm graft. Hemodialysis catheter access was required while he underwent planned right lower extremity hemodialysis graft placement. **A:** A maximum intensity projection (MIP) in the coronal plane using a two-dimensional time-of-flight technique shows a patent left subclavian vein (*arrowhead*), left brachiocephalic vein (*straight arrow*), and SVC (*curved arrow*). A left subclavian vein hemodialysis catheter was successfully inserted. Both internal jugular veins were thrombosed. **B:** An MIP of the inferior vena cava and iliac veins in the coronal plane reveals a widely patent deep venous system. A right thigh graft was successfully placed.

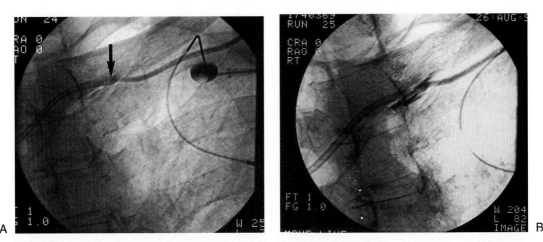

FIG. 3.9. An example of a patient who developed the pinch-off syndrome. The patient had pancreatic cancer. A left subclavian vein Hickman catheter had been inserted surgically several months earlier. The patient now complained of left chest pain with injection of the catheter. **A:** A preliminary scout radiograph demonstrates extrinsic compression of the catheter between the first rib and clavicle (*arrow*). **B:** Contrast extravasation occurs upon catheter injection. In other cases, the catheter may fracture and embolize within the vascular system.

Subclavian Vein Cannulation

The subclavian vein insertion site is approached at a point 1 to 2 cm below the junction of the inner and middle thirds of the clavicle with the needle directed toward the sternal notch. The needle is advanced toward the reference point following a medial and cephalic course with the needle kept almost horizontal to the table. Having the patient perform a Valsalva maneuver or placing the patient in the Trendelenburg position may help distend the vein, facilitating the puncture.

A potential difficulty that can occur with a very medially placed subclavian vein puncture is compression of the catheter by musculoskeletal structures at the confluence of the first rib and clavicle. The compression of the catheter has been termed the pinch-off syndrome and may result in catheter dysfunction, catheter extravasation, or outright catheter fracture (Fig. 3.9) (27).

ACCESS SITES

The chapters that follow address in further detail specific sites used for particular types of vascular access devices. However, it is useful in the assessment of various sites available for use to have a paradigm or framework upon which to select the best site for each particular case at hand.

In general, the right IJV should be considered the primary venous access site for various reasons (28). It is a relatively large, superficially located vein that offers a relatively straight shot to the SVC and RA. The incidence of symptomatic catheter-induced thrombosis or stenosis is lower in the IJV compared with subclavian vein access (29). The incidence of stenoses occurring as a result of subclavian vein access is variably reported but may be as high as 50% (30–33). These findings apply to hemodialysis patients as well as other patients. The right IJV catheter has no effect on intracerebral pressures, and because of the extensive collateral network in the neck, deep venous thrombosis (DVT) of the IJV is well tolerated. The patients do need to be treated for DVT, and pulmonary emboli can occur in such cases (34). The occurrence of stenosis or occlusion secondary to subclavian vein access has led to the recognition by the National Kidney Foundation-sponsored Dialysis Outcomes Quality Initiative (DOQI) that the subclavian vein not be used for CVA in hemodialysis patients (35).

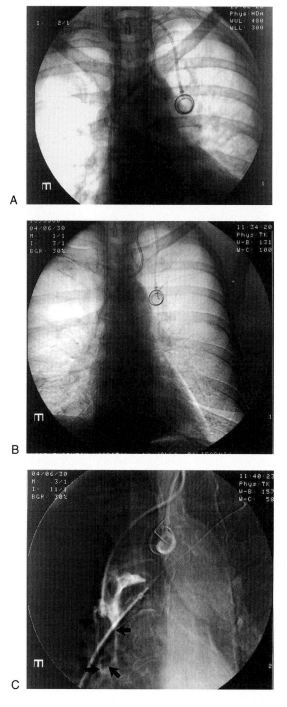

A

B

C

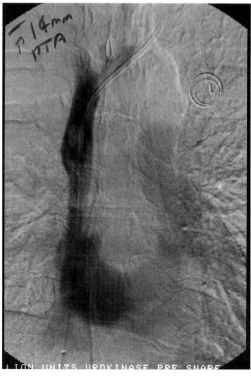

D

FIG. 3.10. The patient is a 65-year-old woman with breast cancer who developed catheter dysfunction after left internal jugular vein portacatheter placement. **A:** The initial postplacement film shows the catheter tip at the right atrium-SVC junction. **B:** The catheter functioned well for approximately 3 months, at which time the nurses were able to infuse but could not aspirate blood from the port. The catheter tip appears to have migrated cephalad several centimeters. **C:** Left anterior oblique projection while the catheter is injected demonstrates a large thrombus (23.4 mm diameter by 89 mm long) extending from the catheter tip (*arrows*). **D:** After 1 million units of urokinase (Abbott Laboratories, N. Chicago, IL, U.S.A.) by pulse spray pharmacomechanical thrombolysis, 14-mm balloon angioplasty, and 25-mm catheter snaring, a marked improvement with function was restored to the portacatheter. The catheter functioned for an additional 3 months and was removed as the patient finished her therapy.

If the right IJV is not available, the left IJV is recommended. Some data suggest, however, that the patency rates are lower with left subclavian vein or left IJV accesses compared with right-sided accesses (29,33) (Fig. 3.10). To minimize clotting using a left-sided approach, care must be taken to have the catheter extend to at least the caval atrial junction or proximal RA. Catheters malpositioned from the left side with the tip near the BCV-SVC junction can cause local venous wall irritation, which may lead to DVT and catheter dysfunction or symptomatic upper extremity swelling.

The subclavian vein access should probably be reserved for select cases. Such cases could include patients with skin conditions precluding use in the neck, patients with occluded IJVs, patients with tracheostomies, patients with prior subclavian vein or BCV stents, or patients who prefer that the access be away from the neck.

In select cases where the conventional sites cannot be used, other sites used for access in rather novel ways include the common femoral veins, inferior vena cava (IVC), hepatic veins, and dilated venous collaterals (see Chapter 12).

Concerning picclines and armports, the favored veins are the basilic veins because these are the most superficial and largest veins. There is also no accompanying artery adjacent to the basilic vein. The cephalic vein is probably the second most used vein, again because it is superficial and has no adjacent artery. The cephalic vein is more difficult to puncture because it is frequently smaller than the basilic vein and is prone to rolling away from the needle. Advancing the catheter from the cephalic vein into the subclavian vein may be difficult due to the entry angle of the cephalic vein with this draining conduit. The brachial veins can be used as well, but these are frequently the smallest and deepest veins available. They are frequently paired and run adjacent to the brachial artery.

IMAGING BASED CVA

Fluoroscopy Guidance for CVA

Techniques have developed that allow access into the subclavian veins and axillary veins using fluoroscopy (36). In this study, the anatomic relationship of the subclavian vein with respect to the first rib was determined using venograms in 42 patients. The study determined that the subclavian vein typically crossed the radial segment of the first rib at 94.7 ± 7.4 degrees (mean ± standard deviation) (Fig. 3.11). The vein projects approximately 5 degrees inferior to the most lateral portion of the first rib with respect to the interpedicular line. The investigators attempted 42 punctures using fluoroscopy alone and achieved success in all cases with an average of 2.9 passes. Most cases required fewer passes (skewed distribution with a few outliers with many passes), because the median number of passes was only 1.7. The authors had a 5% complication rate due to subclavian artery punctures (both with unusual caudally positioned subclavian veins).

The skin entry site in the infraclavicular fossa is determined fluoroscopically, 3 to 4 cm lateral and just caudal to the most lateral point of the first rib. Local anesthesia is infiltrated medially toward the first rib. A 7 cm long, 21-gauge needle (Cook Inc., Bloomington, IN, U.S.A.) is passed along this tract at a fairly shallow angle until the needle tip projects over the lateral margin of the first rib (Fig. 3.12). The needle angle is adjusted such that the tip is

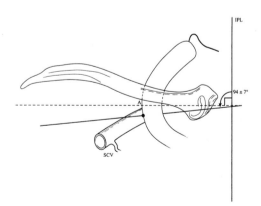

FIG. 3.11. Diagram demonstrating usual location of the subclavian vein with respect to the first rib. A perpendicular from the interpedicular line (*IPL*) crosses the lateralmost portion of the first rib at point A. The subclavian vein is most often found 4 degrees inferior to this point.

made to firmly strike the first rib. Slow withdrawal of the needle with continuous aspiration provides evidence of venous entry. Contrast injection is then made to confirm the central venous entry prior to catheter insertion. The advantages of this method are that it is quick, it does not rely on US equipment (which may not be readily available), the risk of pneumothorax is very low because the puncture is lateral and directed toward a rib and not the lung, and the lateral puncture eliminates possible pinch-off syndrome. The disadvantages of this method are that patency is not established before attempted puncture and the operator may receive radiation to the hand during the final needle advancement. Note that the authors recommend that patients with multiple prior CVAs be scanned preliminarily with US to ensure patency of the planned access route.

In cases in which landmarks or the above method have not been successful, an alternative method consists of fluoroscopic guidance after transfemoral guidewire or catheter placement into the subclavian vein (37). The guidewire or catheter is then used as a target so that the subclavian vein puncture can be performed. The technique also can be used when there is segmental subclavian vein occlusion with reconstitution of the medial subclavian vein segment by collateral veins. Retrograde catheterization of

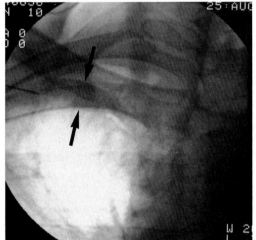

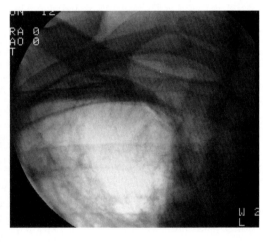

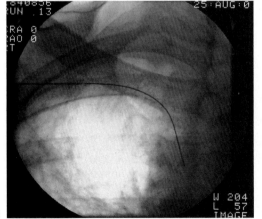

FIG. 3.12. An example of a fluoroscopic right subclavian vein puncture performed with venographic assistance. **A:** Contrast venography in this case via the right upper extremity shows the relationship of the right subclavian vein (*arrows*) to the lateral margin of the first rib. The needle enters the skin 3 to 4 cm more lateral than the lateral margin of the first rib. **B:** The needle is oriented more perpendicular, such that the tip hits the anterior surface of the first rib, thus puncturing the subclavian vein (here outlined by venography) and not the lung. **C:** Successful guidewire advancement after needle puncture of the subclavian vein.

the subclavian veins or axillary veins may be difficult because of the presence of venous valves; the utility of this technique to access the IJVs has not been studied.

Fluoroscopy with Contrast Venography for Central Venous Access

Preferably, a peripheral IV catheter is placed in the median basilic vein within the antecubital fossa (37). If this is not available, another site will suffice. A preliminary venogram (with or without tourniquets) may determine the presence of peripheral or central occlusions important for planning the procedure. A site for preparation and draping is then selected.

The technique for contrast venographic-directed puncture is particularly useful for insertion of picclines and arm ports in the upper extremities (Fig. 3.13). The arm is positioned in abduction with external rotation (supination). Patients unable to maintain this position for the

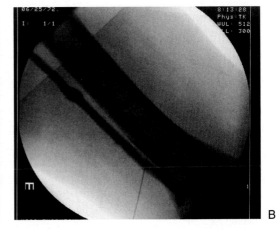

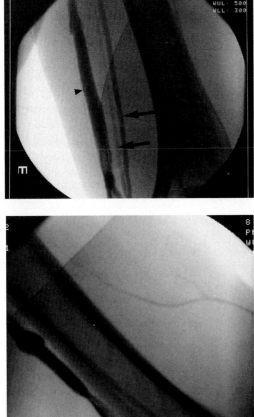

FIG. 3.13. Example of contrast venography to facilitate piccline placement. **A:** A preliminary venogram is performed to outline patency of the upper arm veins. Complete filling, especially of the deeper veins, may be augmented by placing a tourniquet near the axilla. Palpation over the inner aspect of the upper arm during the venogram with a Kelly clamp may help determine the most superficial vein. Note that the brachial vein, which is the most superficial vein, is larger than the deeper, paired brachial veins. **B:** The operator attempts to align the needle (*arrow*) colinear with the vein. In this particular case, the brachial vein is slightly medial to the needle. **C:** Upon imminent puncture of the vein, the contrast column appears less dense, and at puncture blood will aspirate freely, at which point the guidewire can be advanced.

time required for the procedure can be aided by placing a bolster beneath the arm with tape fixation as required. A tourniquet may aid to distend the vein and keep the contrast in place during the puncture, thus reducing the overall volume of contrast needed for the procedure. The middle third of the arm is the desired site of puncture because the piccline hubs need room external to the arm above the elbow to allow flexion to occur freely. A preliminary venogram helps to identify potential obstacles to insertion such as vasospasm, thrombus, or stenoses (38).

The patient is prepared and draped, and repeat venography with tourniquets is performed. Care is taken to not infuse lidocaine too close to the vein because this may cause venospasm (38). Careful coning and magnification fluoroscopy facilitates entry into the contrast-distended vein. A 21-gauge microaccess set is used along with a 0.018-inch guidewire (Coaxial micropuncture introducer set, Cook) to gain access to the vein. With the access needle visualized in the lower portion of the coned, magnified image, the needle is aligned with the longitudinal axis of the desired vein (Fig. 3.13). Imminent venous puncture is seen by thinning of the contrast column as the anterior wall of the vein is displaced posteriorly by the advancing needle. The needle is carefully advanced while an assistant applies suction through extension tubing. Once a flash of blood is seen, the assistant should notify the operator immediately. The operator often feels a characteristic pop as the needle punctures the resistance of the venous wall. If free blood can be aspirated, the tubing can be carefully disconnected and the guidewire advanced. It is not unusual to create a double-wall puncture, in which case blood will not aspirate freely. In this case, it is best to lower the needle hub toward the skin, which helps to align the needle with the axis of the vein. While suction is applied, the needle is very slowly withdrawn until blood appears. If no blood is aspirated, or the guidewire could not be advanced, repuncture is often required, with an attempt made to puncture a little more cephalad on the arm. Occasionally, the guidewire hangs up at the tourniquet location, which should then be released. More lidocaine is then

given, and, if needed, the needle entry site can be widened with a no. 11 blade (Bard Parker, Franklin Lakes, NJ, U.S.A.) and a curved Kelly clamp. The peel-away sheath is advanced. The guidewire is often used to estimate the catheter length so that the piccline can be cut to the exact dimensions required to reach the SVC-RA junction.

Although fluoroscopic puncture of the subclavian vein can be performed in the majority of cases, it is limited in cases where central vein stenosis or occlusions may occur (36). Moreover, another venographic study performed by Yeow and colleagues (39) documented that in 11% of 280 patients, access to the subclavian vein over the anterior aspect of the first rib was obstructed by the clavicle. In these cases, the investigators were able to access the axillary vein over the second rib rather than the first. Preliminary venograms were performed. In cases where access to the subclavian vein was precluded, a 21-gauge needle 7 cm long (Coaxial micropuncture introducer set, Cook) attached to a syringe with vacuum was used to access the axillary vein over the second rib. The preliminary run was stored on a second screen to aid the puncture, and using careful coning the needle advanced toward the anterior second rib. Occasionally additional small amounts of contrast were given to help localize the axillary vein. The needle was advanced until blood was aspirated or the bone was reached. If no blood return occurred, the needle was slowly withdrawn with gentle suction. When free blood flow occurred, a 0.018-inch guidewire was advanced to the RA. Using this method in 31 cases, the operators achieved access with an average of 1.5 needle passes. There were no instances of pneumothorax or arterial punctures, and no nerve injuries occurred. The average contrast load was approximately 50 mL. One disadvantage of this method is that the axillary vein is slightly deeper than the subclavian vein, which may result in a steeper angle made between the introducer sheath and the vein, which may result in a kinked sheath through which the catheter cannot be advanced.

Other variations using contrast venograms to obtain subclavian vein access have included a standard fluoroscopically guided Seldinger technique with a preceding "road map" (40), venography performed with the image intensifier positioned with approximately 30 degrees of caudal angulation (41), and venopuncture performed over the first rib during venography with the tube in a 25 degree anterior oblique position (42).

Ultrasonographic Guidance for Central Venous Access

Ultrasonography is currently our method of choice for obtaining CVA either in the neck, chest, or periphery. The advantages include the ability to visualize the veins and arteries in real time, allowing assessment of important variants in anatomic positioning of these structures that potentially limit landmark-based methods. Some of the disadvantages of the venographic approach is the requirement for a peripheral IV, the requirement for iodinated contrast with risks of allergic reactions and nephrotoxicity, and the additional radiation exposure to the operator and patient needed with venography. The direct visualization of the needle and vein minimizes the chances for pneumothorax or arterial punctures. Although access can be made with real-time US, the addition of color or gated Doppler allows clear identification of artery versus vein. Moreover, the Doppler data provide useful information, which helps predict the success of that particular planned access site. The large dilated vein visualized with real-time US may be present because of a more central venous stenosis or occlusion. The utility of the Doppler examination is underscored in the hemodialysis or oncology patient who returns not infrequently for new CVAs.

Ultrasonographic Guidance into the Internal Jugular Veins and Subclavian Veins

Internal Jugular Vein Access

Central venoocclusive disease of the neck and chest is increasing in frequency because of the wide scale application of CVA (43–45). Secondary to the development of extensive collateral networks, slowly progressive central venous occlusion is often well tolerated and may be asymptomatic (44,46). It has been demonstrated that in such asymptomatic patients, sonographic imaging alone misses most cases of central venoocclusive disease (47). A total of 67 patients were studied, all of whom were presently asymptomatic, although five had previous histories of upper extremity swelling. The patients underwent both duplex US evaluation of the axillary veins and IJVs and contrast venography before CVA. Duplex evaluation included visual evidence of venoocclusive disease as well as presence or absence of normal transmitted polyphasic RA waves and respiratory variation of flow. Direct sonographic imaging of the axillary veins and IJVs allowed detection of access route venoocclusive disease with a sensitivity of only 33%. However, when Doppler flow analysis found that RA waveforms were not polyphasic, central occlusive disease was detected with a sensitivity of 79.6% (Fig. 3.4). Moreover, monophasic RA waveforms were associated with a 25% failure rate of catheterization secondary to central vein occlusion. In contrast, polyphasic RA waveforms were associated with a 100% success rate for CVA. The presence of a polyphasic RA waveform virtually excludes the possibility of a more central venous occlusion or stenosis greater than 80%. Approximately half of the patient population had risk factors for central venous disease, including patients with prior central lines, hemodialysis accesses, mediastinal tumors or adenopathy, irradiation, or pacemakers. The influence of these risk factors on the venographic findings is illustrated in Tables 3.2 and 3.3. All the patients with a history of upper extremity swelling suffered from stenoses greater than 80% (one case) or occlusions (four cases).

The superficial location of the IJV makes it ideally suited for US evaluation. Before the patient is prepared and draped, an examination of the vein in transverse and longitudinal planes is performed. Next, flow is assessed with color and gated Doppler examinations; this is best performed with the transducer oriented in a longitudinal plane. The patient is prepared and

TABLE 3.2. *The influence of various risk factors upon venographic findings of central conduit disease*

Patient cohort*	Venographic findings		
	Normal	30%–99% stenosis	Occlusion
(+) RFs	31.4%	40%	28.6%
(−) RFs	77.8%	22.2%	0%

RF, risk factors: prior central line, hemodialysis access, radiation therapy, mediastinal tumor or adenopathy, pacemaker.

draped, and the US probe (either 5 or 7.5 MHz) is placed in a sterile cover. A 21-gauge microaccess needle 7 cm long (Coaxial micropuncture introducer set) is connected to a 12- or 20-mL syringe with connector tubing. Alternatively, a standard 18-gauge single-wall needle (Remington Medical Inc., Alpharetta, GA, U.S.A.) can be used for the puncture. Specially designed needles with added surface irregularity are available at increased cost versus conventional needles, which offer greater needle conspicuity on US; but usually the standard needles can be well visualized by careful sweeping of the US probe combined with gentle to-and-fro motion of the needle.

The IJV can be entered in one of two ways (28) (Fig 3.14). The first method has been referred to as the low approach, which actually corresponds with the middle approach referred to earlier when discussing the traditional puncture methods (48). The vein is accessed between the sternal and clavicular heads of the sternocleidomastoid muscle. The advantages of this method are that it avoids hitting the EJV during the puncture or tunneling. Access through the SCM muscle is avoided, which may decrease the risk of bleeding. Lastly, the low IJV puncture facilitates creation of a gently curved catheter course from the IJV to the skin exit site.

With the low approach, the probe is held transverse to the vein at the base of the neck and pressure is applied with a finger or Kelly clamp along the middle of the transducer to identify a site in close proximity to the vein. Anesthesia is applied with 1% lidocaine (Abbott Laboratories, N. Chicago, IL, U.S.A.) at that site only to the superficial tissues. Care must be maintained to not inject air into the subcutaneous tissues, which limits the effectiveness of US. The access needle is then directed at the IJV. The needle is advanced with continuous suction applied; the pathway of needle advancement is such as to project a pathway colinear with the expected path of the IJV. This facilitates guidewire advancement once venous entry occurs. Sweeping the transducer cephalocaudal simultaneously with to-and-fro motion of the needle facilitates needle tip visualization. When the needle tip is near the superficial aspect of the vein, the soft tissues near the venous wall move with the to-and-fro needle motion and the patient may indicate that he or she is feeling a sharp sensation. At this point the needle is carefully advanced, and often a characteristic pop is felt. The blood flow from the needle sometimes is brisk, indicating successful puncture. More often, only a flash in the needle hub or tubing is noted. The procedure is based on two active participants: the operator advances the needle and observes the US monitor, and the assistant provides suction and observes for blood return. In the case of blood flashback, displacement of

TABLE 3.3. *Range of stenoses found in the study population*

	Percent diameter stenosis on venography		
	30%–40%	50%–79%	80%–99%
35 patients with stenoses	10	20	5

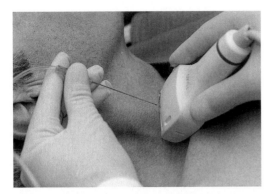

FIG. 3.14. There are two methods commonly used to puncture the internal jugular vein (IJV) via ultrasonography (US). In the majority of cases, the IJV is located anterolateral or lateral to the common carotid artery (CCA). In these cases, the IJV can be punctured by orienting the US transducer perpendicular to the vein and puncturing the vein with the needle directed near the mid-point of the transducer held such that the IJV is in the middle of the field of view. Care must be taken to not compress the vein by the weight of the transducer. Sweeping the transducer superiorly to inferiorly while the needle is moved to and fro allows visualization of the needle tip with respect to the IJV, aiding in puncture placement. Note that if a two-wall puncture is created through the IJV, the CCA is not violated.

If the vein is difficult to visualize, additional maneuvers such as positioning the head flat (without a pillow) and turned away from the site of puncture will flatten the subcutaneous tissues and give more room to work. A variety of factors increase the IJV size, the most effective being the Trendelenburg position, an abdominal binder, and the Valsalva maneuver (26). In the study by Armstrong and colleagues, 35 US studies of normal volunteers demonstrated that the average IJV diameter was 11.5 mm. There was a poor correlation between neck size (r = 0.22), age (r = 0.36), height (r = -0.23), or weight (r = 0.10), and IJV size. The IJV was anterior to the carotid artery in 2 cases, anterolateral in 12, and lateral in 21. Too forceful a compression of the vein with the transducer also may collapse the vein.

In the second IJV access method (Fig. 3.15), also performed with the transducer transverse to the needle, the needle access is lined up with the long axis of the transducer, generally just above the clavicle. This approach uses a lateral approach to the vein, which has two advantages. Occasionally, the CCA is directly beneath the IJV (0.3%) (28), and the above method risks simultaneous venous and arterial

the needle down toward the skin and slow and careful removal of the needle (so that it remains parallel with the IJV) with simultaneous suction will elicit blood return. A guidewire is then advanced under fluoroscopic control. It is useful to have the pulse monitor at an audible level to help inform the operator whether these guidewire maneuvers are eliciting atrial or ventricular ectopy.

The larger 18-gauge single-wall access needle readily reveals the pulsatile nature of an inadvertent arterial puncture, whereas the smaller 21-gauge needle may only elicit a prominent dribble, which may be indeterminate as to which structure has been punctured. Advancement of the guidewire into the IVC will confirm for the operator that a venous puncture has occurred in cases where an artery may have been punctured. Cases where the artery has been punctured are managed by removal and compression.

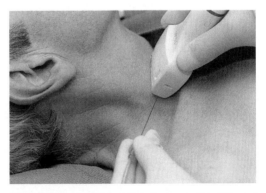

FIG. 3.15. In a minority of cases, the internal jugular vein (IJV) is directly anterior to the common carotid artery (CCA). In these cases, the approach to the IJV is different. The transducer is held in a similar fashion, perpendicular to the vein, and the puncture is performed from a lateral approach. In this case, if a two-wall IJV puncture is performed, the CCA is avoided.

punctures, as well as arterial venous fistula formation. The lateral approach avoids this. In addition, the lateral approach facilitates tunneling the catheter out to the lateral chest wall.

Once access has been obtained, the 0.018-inch guidewire can be advanced so that the wire tip lies at the desired location. Next, the intravascular length is determined for cuffed catheters that cannot be cut to fit (dialysis catheters) (49). A clamp is placed on the hub end of the guidewire and the exact intravascular length of the guidewire is determined by subtracting the extravascular length of the catheter. Knowing the intravascular length of the catheter determines the length needed for the tunnel for proper positioning of the cuff. The cuff should be placed 2 to 3 cm above the catheter exit site. After tunneling, the 0.018-inch guidewire is replaced with a standard 0.035-inch guidewire and a peel-away sheath is inserted.

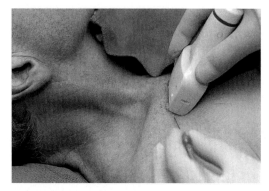

FIG. 3.16. The ultrasonographic (US) approach to the subclavian vein is facilitated by orienting the transducer along the longitudinal axis of the subclavian vein. The needle is advanced under direct US visualization at the lateral margin of the US transducer toward the vein until blood can be aspirated from the needle.

Subclavian Vein Access

Although imaging the subclavian vein in a sagittal direction may readily help distinguish the vein (larger diameter, more superficial and caudal position) from the artery, accessing the subclavian vein is best performed with the long axis of the transducer aligned with the vein. The subclavian vein is accessed more laterally than with landmark methods so that the pinch-off syndrome is avoided (27). In general, the puncture is started at about the subcoracoid location or medially with the needle at a 30 degree angle with respect to the skin. The longitudinal orientation of the needle along the long axis of the transducer facilitates needle tip visualization in contrast to the transversely oriented probe used to puncture the IJV (Fig. 3.16). The needle is advanced, checking needle tip location with similar maneuvers as described above, and puncture occurs again with a characteristic pop sensation. The lateral approach to the subclavian vein reduces the pneumothorax risk because the distance to the pleura is increased. Moreover, the artery and vein become further separated the more lateral the puncture is performed. If a very medial puncture is performed, for example, as medial as with the landmark

method, particularly if the patient is cachectic, the pleura and lung may be directly opposed. A double-wall puncture of the vein in this case may result in a pneumothorax. If air is returned through the flushed needle or extension tubing while attempting to puncture the vein, a possible pneumothorax may be occurring.

Ultrasonographic Puncture of Peripheral Veins

Ultrasonography is ideally suited for creation of piccline or arm port accesses. Before the patient is prepared, the nondominant arm is examined with a 7.5-MHz linear US probe. The vein is examined by compression to exclude thrombus or an artery. The use of tourniquets helps to distend the vein, making access potentially easier, but may make compression maneuvers or Doppler examination more difficult to interpret. In a patient with a prior history of CVA, a quick look at the ipsilateral axillary vein and subclavian vein may help indicate if problems exist in the more central conduits (47).

After a site has been chosen, typically above the elbow, the tourniquet is applied and the arm scanned with the US transducer oriented transverse to the vein. When a suitable vein has been localized, the spot directly over the vein is anesthetized with 1% lidocaine. This is easily performed by sliding a Kelly clamp beneath the transducer face; at the point where the shadow from the clamp obscures the vein, the anesthetic is applied. A 21-gauge, 7-cm needle (Coaxial micropuncture introducer set) is connected to tubing and a syringe to apply suction. The needle is advanced and the needle tip is sought again with a to-and-fro or wiggling motion of the needle and back-and-forth scanning with the US transducer. When the needle tip is seen directly on top of the vein, a relatively quick thrust with the needle is made. As with other venous accesses, the puncture is felt as a characteristic pop; the puncture is often of the double-wall type. Dropping the needle hub closer to the skin, aligning the needle with the expected orientation of the vein, and slow withdrawal of the needle provide blood return. The 0.018-inch guidewire can then be advanced. If difficulty is encountered with advancement of the guidewire, careful movement of the needle and probing with the guidewire may allow advancement of the guidewire, much as in approaching a common femoral artery puncture. Sometimes the needle must be pulled back minimally to allow the guidewire to be advanced. Occasionally, the guidewire does not advance past the tourniquet, which is easily resolved by releasing the tension. Unlike central veins, the peripheral veins may develop spasm, limiting passage of the guidewire or catheter. Venospasm can occasionally be treated with nitroglycerin (100 µg IV; Abbott) (50).

Once guidewire access is obtained, the peelaway sheath is inserted. The guidewire can be used to estimate the length of the catheter for picclines in a method similar to that described earlier for dialysis catheters.

COMPARISON OF TRADITIONAL LANDMARK AND IMAGE-GUIDED METHODS OF CENTRAL VENOUS ACCESS

The landmark methods of CVA are typically favored in the mainstream, particularly among surgeons. These methods are cheap and quick, and have been considered effective for several decades. However, IJV and subclavian vein puncture requires the position of a deep vein to be identified with surface landmarks. Hence, the precise location of the vein is unknown, and it is usually impossible to detect venous occlusion or anomaly. Certain factors such as physician experience have been recognized as important factors in the success of landmark methods for catheterization. Inability to insert catheters with landmark methods into specific veins has occurred in up to 19% of IJV attempts and approximately 12% of subclavian vein attempts (51). Complication rates have varied with definitions but are reported at 1% to 10% and 0.3% to 12% for IJV and subclavian vein attempts, respectively (Figs. 3.17–3.19). Numerous studies have demonstrated the benefit of percutaneous methods over cutdown with respect to reduced complications such as bleeding and hematoma and decreased failures and catheter malpositions. One large, retrospective study looked specifically at landmark methods to obtain large-bore catheter access using either the IJV or subclavian vein (52). The study involved 2,741 catheters in 1,216 patients, with 2,179 accessed by the IJV and 562 accessed by the subclavian vein. Complications were more frequent with the subclavian vein approach

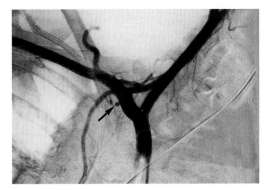

FIG. 3.17. The patient is an elderly woman who developed a right neck and chest hematoma after placement of a right subclavian vein catheter. The angiogram of the right subclavian artery demonstrates a pseudoaneurysm (*arrow*) along the inferior aspect of the artery just medial to the internal mammary artery. The pseudoaneurysm was repaired surgically.

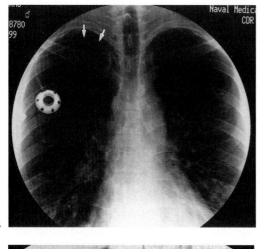

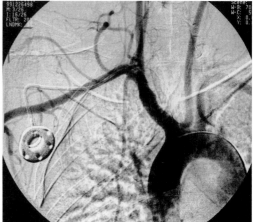

A

B

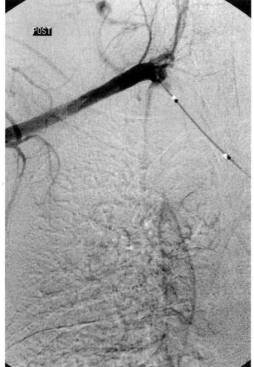

C

FIG. 3.18. The patient is a 38-year-old man with metastatic carcinoma of the rectum. **A:** The patient had a surgically placed right chest porta-catheter that was causing transient ischemic attacks each time the port was flushed. The spot radiography shows the anomalously high position of the catheter (*arrows*) above the clavicle. The subclavian vein does not normally extend this cephalad. **B:** A right subclavian arteriogram demonstrates the catheter entering the right subclavian artery. **C:** The catheter was successfully removed with a balloon catheter positioned nearby if vascular control could not be obtained by manual compression alone. (Case courtesy of T. Velling, M.D.)

(48.9%) than with the IJV approach (24.8%). The IJV had lower failure rates (0.4%) and less bleeding (1.1%) and no pneumothoraces compared with the subclavian vein route: 4.5% failures, 2.7% bleeding, 3.2% pneumothorax/hemothorax. A higher arterial puncture rate was noted with IJV (4.3%) than with subclavian vein (1.4%) punctures. Lower infection rates were noted with IJV punctures (8.8%) than with subclavian vein (15.3%) punctures.

Although the clinical utility of imaging guidance to obtain CVA is readily apparent to interventionalists who perform venous access on a daily basis, not all reports favor imaging. For example, Mansfield et al. reported on a prospective, randomized study of subclavian vein catheterization in 821 patients, of which 411 were performed with US assistance and 410 were performed with traditional landmark methods (51). A significant limitation of the

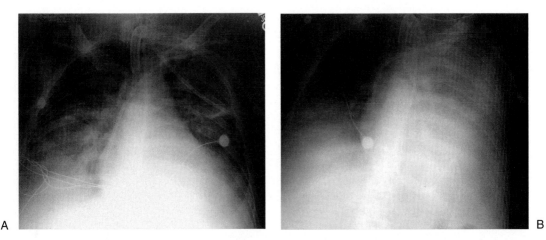

FIG. 3.19. A 43-year-old male liver transplant patient needed hemodialysis. **A:** A left subclavian vein hemodialysis catheter was placed surgically. **B:** The patient developed a large left pleural effusion 4 days after line placement, which upon chest tube insertion was revealed to be a chylothorax (high pleural fluid triglycerides). The chyle leak resolved with conservative treatment.

study is that US was used only to measure the depth and caliber of the subclavian vein at the level of the clavicle, determine its patency, and mark its location on the skin. Access was then performed in a conventional fashion. Real-time US guidance was not used for creation of the access. US and landmark methods resulted in similar subclavian vein catheterization failures and complications in 12.4% versus 12% and 9.7% versus 9.8%, respectively. Despite the limitations of this study concerning the use of US, the study did identify a group of patients at high risk for failure and acute complications. Failed attempts were twice as likely in patients who were especially thin or obese or who had previously undergone major surgery or CVA (14.2% vs. 8.1%). Prior surgery or radiation therapy was hypothesized to cause slight shifting of the position of the subclavian vein or an alternation of the surface landmarks used to locate the vein. A failed catheterization attempt was the strongest predictor of a subsequent complication. Complications included arterial puncture (3.7%), pneumothorax (1.5%), and mediastinal hematoma (0.6%). These complications occurred in approximately one fourth of the patients in whom the subclavian vein catheterization was unsuccessful. Mansfield et al. believe the DVT rate to be higher with the left-sided accesses compared with right accesses (51). A second prospective study of the landmark method in 150 consecutive infraclav-

TABLE 3.4. *The results of randomized trials comparing landmark methods and ultrasonography to obtain access into the IJVs*

Investigator	Cases (n)	Success[a] (%)	First try[b] (%)	Time(s)	CA puncture[c] (%)	Brach plexus[d] (%)	Hematoma (%)
Denys (54)	302/302	88/100	38/78	45/10	8.3/1.7	1.7/0.4	3.3/0.2
Teich (55)	50/50	N/R	52/96	51/15	12/0	6/4	10/2

Values represent landmark method/ultrasonographic method.
[a]Percentage of patients who were successfully catheterized.
[b]Percentage of patients who were accessed on the first needle pass.
[c]Percentage of patients in whom the carotid artery was punctured.
[d]Percentage of patients who had irritation of the brachial plexus.
[e]Percentage of patients who got hematomas.
N/R, not reported.

icular subclavian vein accesses demonstrated a higher complication rate using the right subclavian vein (35.5%) compared with the left (12.5%) (p < 0.01) (53). The largest share of complications from the right side related to arterial punctures (9.1% vs. 0% from the left).

Two studies have analyzed prospective, randomized trials of landmark methods versus real-time US for venous access via the IJVs (54,55). Both studies concluded that US-guided cannulation of the IJV significantly improved success rates, decreased access times, and decreased complication rates (Table 3.4).

IMAGING TO SOLVE SPECIFIC INSERTION PROBLEMS

One advantage available to interventionalists inserting central venous catheters in comparison with our surgical colleagues is the ability to recognize malpositioned lines and make immediate corrections. In general, the right IJV represents a straight shot to the RA and SVC. The only possible vein that may mimic the SVC on anteroposterior fluoroscopy is the azygous vein (Fig. 3.20). If doubt remains, oblique fluoroscopy or contrast injection will immediately provide clarification. Prevention is probably the best course, and careful observation of the 0.018-inch or 0.035-inch guidewire as it is advanced from the BCV into the SVC to the RA and IVC may help indicate whether improper selection has occurred. In general, a guidewire does not pass as easily into the smaller azygous vein, or the loop in the guidewire (if a floppy J guidewire is used) appears abnormally small compared with that expected for either the SVC or IVC. Once the operator is sure of the guidewire location, it is probably best to keep the guidewire at that location; for example, if the guidewire is pulled way cephalad before insertion of the sheath, the azygous vein may be inadvertently selected without the operator realizing it. If a right subclavian vein puncture has been performed, the guidewire and catheter may be misplaced into the opposite BCV or subclavian vein because the needle or sheath may point directly in this direction. This is easily redirected with an angled Glidewire (Medi-Tech/

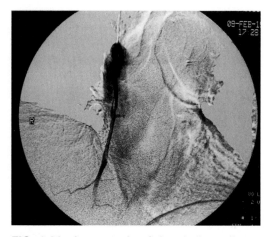

FIG. 3.20. An example of the similar pathway taken by the SVC and azygous vein as seen on anteroposterior fluoroscopy. In this case, an attempt was made to place a hemodialysis catheter. The operator recognized that advancement of the guidewire was limited upon trying to advance the guidewire into the inferior vena cava. An injection was then performed, revealing the aberrant catheterization, which was corrected, and the hemodialysis catheter was inserted without difficulty.

Boston Scientific, Watertown, MA, U.S.A.). Alternatively, the catheter can be manipulated with a tip-deflecting wire (Cook) (56). Malpositioning of catheters inserted from left-sided punctures is less common than from the right because of the angles that the left BCV make with the SVC compared with those from the right.

Occasionally, despite successful guidewire insertion, the operator has difficulty advancing the peel-away sheath. Careful assessment by visual as well as fluoroscopic methods may help indicate the problem. Rarely, fatal complications have occurred by careless attempts at advancement of the peel-away sheath (57). The hypothesized link leading to these complications appears to be kinking of the guidewire that occurs outside the venous entry site or at a site of severe angulation within the vein. The kink becomes the leading edge of the advancing dilator, resulting in either a tear in the venous entry site or a perforation more centrally. This is avoided by careful control of the guidewire during insertion of the sheath under fluoroscopy. If the guidewire is kinked, it should be removed and replaced with a new and preferably stiffer one. An inadequate skin nick or one with a bridge of crossing soft tissue is detected by buckling of the skin with forward pressure on the sheath. This is solved by careful use of a no. 10 scalpel blade (Bard Parker, Franklin Lakes, NJ) and curved Kelly clamps. Alternatively, the problem may be deeper in the tissues of the neck or chest, particularly in patients who have had CVAs before. Fluoroscopy may help to vectorally align the guidewire and sheath in a colinear path so that force is efficiently transferred to the entry site. The operator should try to resist pushing too hard on the peel-away sheath: raising an edge on the sheath may make its advancement more difficult and possibly traumatize the venous wall, resulting in bleeding. It may be advantageous to use a stiffer wire. Inserting the dilator only from the peel-away sheath set often works, particularly if time is allowed for tissue viscoelastic relaxation. Overdilatation may work but may increase the pericatheter oozing that may occur. If the sheath is not usable, using another peel-away sheath is often helpful because the sheaths supplied with the catheter are often inferior in quality to what is available in the interventionalist's supply.

Another problem that can occur is sheath kinking, which precludes catheter insertion despite initial successful guidewire insertion. The kinked sheath compromises the luminal diameter of the sheath sufficiently that the catheter cannot be advanced owing to the low column strength of current grade silicon catheters. Robertson et al. reported that kinked sheaths occur because of acute angulations—either where the sheath enters the vein or more centrally, or because of extrinsic compression of the sheath by venous stenoses or beneath the clavicle (58).

In the case of the compressed sheath, the sheath may appear normal fluoroscopically while supported by the inner dilator but collapses once the dilator is removed and attempts are made to advance the catheter, carefully advancing a Glidewire through one lumen of the catheter into the IVC and removal of the peel-away sheath/catheter maintains access. A conventional vascular sheath can be inserted and the problem outlined by contrast injection. The stenosis can be dilated with conventional techniques, at which point catheter reinsertion can be attempted with a new peel-away sheath.

Kinking related to acute angulations are solved by different methods. If the kink occurs well beyond the venous access site, careful withdrawal of the sheath so that the kink can be straightened may allow the catheter to be advanced. The pushability of the soft silastic catheter can be augmented by inserting a guidewire (or two guidewires for two-lumen catheters) (Medi-tech/Boston Scientific). Kinking of the sheath at the venous entry site is often a technical problem related to how the venopuncture was performed. In general, the more perpendicular the access is created with respect to the vein, the more likely that sheath kinking will be a problem. Occasionally, inserting a different but similar sized peel-away sheath solves this problem, as discussed earlier. Alternatively, attempting to change the position of the upper extremity or overdilating the venous tract may work (58). Robertson et al. resorted to leaving a vascular dilator in the vessel overnight as one method to insert a vascular sheath the following day (58). Another maneuver that we have used occasionally, is to carefully advance a Glidewire into each lumen through the kink into the entry vein and then on to the IVC. The wires are fixed to the catheter by flow switches (Medi-tech/Boston Scientific). The sheath is removed, and the catheters are carefully advanced along with the guidewires to the proper position (Fig. 3.21).

The last serious problem that can occur during attempted catheter insertion through a peel-away sheath is air embolism (Fig. 3.22) (59). This can lead to serious complications and even death. In general, it is far better to take the necessary steps to prevent this complication rather than deal with the stresses and compromises (sterile technique) in treating this condition. The appearance of air embolism provides a rather dramatic fluoroscopic image not easily forgotten with air seen in the right ventricle, pulmonary outflow tract, and pulmonary arter-

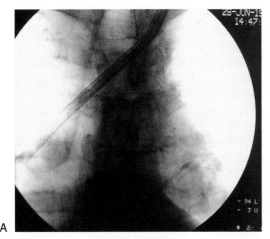

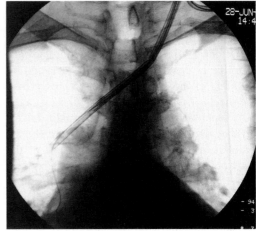

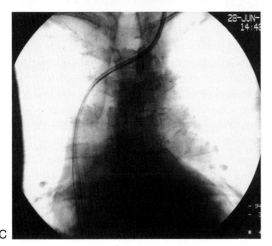

FIG. 3.21. An example of the inability to advance a double-lumen catheter because of sheath kinking. **A:** The catheter could only be partially advanced through the sheath, which enters via a left internal jugular vein approach. **B:** A stiff Glidewire has been advanced through the catheter, which is secured to the hub end of the catheter with the aid of a flow valve placed over the guidewire and closed. Next, the catheter and guidewire are carefully held in place while the peel-away sheath is removed. **C:** With the kinked sheath removed, the catheter can easily be advanced to the proper location.

ies. Preventive maneuvers include Trendelenburg positioning or instructing the patient to exhale or hum while the catheter is being inserted. The sheath also can be crimped between the fingers, or saline can be flushed through the lumen of the advancing end of the catheter as it enters the sheath. This last maneuver ensures that fluid enters the sheath rather than air. Having a saline-soaked gauze or telfa pad (Kendal Co., Mansfield, MA, U.S.A.) nearby can be useful to act as an improvised seal against the end of the sheath in difficult cases.

Rapid entry of a large volume of air puts a strain on the right ventricle because of migration of air to the pulmonary circulation. The pulmonary artery pressures increase and the pulmonary vascular return decreases, which diminishes left ventricular preload. This decreases the cardiac output so that cardiovascular collapse may occur. Tachyarrhythmias and bradyarrhythmias also may occur. When large quantities of gas (>50 cc) are injected abruptly, acute cor pulmonale, asystole, or both are likely to occur. This altered vascular resistance of the pulmonary arteries results in ventilation perfusion (V/Q) mismatch, resulting in right-to-left shunting and increased alveolar dead space, causing arterial hypoxia and hypercapnea.

To treat air embolism, further gas entry must be stopped. In certain cases, therapy with catecholamines is required, as is cardiopulmonary resuscitation. Adequate oxygenation is often

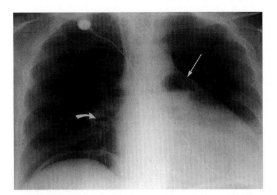

FIG. 3.22. The patient is a 52-year-old woman with a perforated duodenal ulcer who underwent portable chest radiography after central line placement preoperatively. A large amount of air is seen in the main pulmonary artery (*straight arrow*) and right pulmonary arteries (*curved arrow*) on this upright film. In this case, the patient was asymptomatic and treated conservatively.

possible with an increase in oxygen concentration of the inspired gas (up to 100%). This favors the exit of nitrogen gas from the pulmonary capillaries by a favorable gradient. Catheterization of the right ventricle or pulmonary arteries can be attempted. Occasional reports have recommend right-side-up positioning, although one source recommended supine positioning (59).

IMAGING FOR PROPER CATHETER POSITIONING

Historically CVA devices were placed using anatomic landmarks for venipuncture. Postprocedural chest radiographs were used to determine the course of the catheter and the position of the catheter tip and to exclude procedural complications such as pneumothorax or mediastinal hemorrhage. With the use of various imaging techniques through the procedure by interventional radiologists, the need to perform routine postprocedural radiographs has been called into question (60,61). Chang and co-workers reported a retrospective study of 424 patients who underwent 572 IJV catheter insertions (60). The added benefit and estimated costs of postoperative inspiratory and expiratory chest radiographs were studied. US was the method used to obtain access in each case. These investigators found that none of the routine postprocedural chest radiographs revealed a complication not already revealed by routine fluoroscopy. Interestingly, two patients developed symptomatic pneumothoraces (one at 4 hours and the other at 7 hours postprocedure), both of which were not seen, even retrospectively on the postprocedural radiographs. The estimated Medicare reimbursement for the radiographs was a total of $39,559.52 or $34.58 per chest radiograph, films that yielded no useful information.

A second study of the utility of routine chest radiography after central line insertion was reported by Lucey and co-workers (61). A total of 612 catheters were inserted in 489 patients. Various sites were used for access, including 425 right IJVs, 133 left IJVs, and 63 subclavian veins. The vast majority of catheters were for hemodialysis. Intraprocedural fluoroscopy revealed inappropriate catheter tip position or catheter kinks in 90 catheters, all of which were rectified at the time of the procedure. The postprocedural chest radiographs showed no complications, and in only 6 of 621 catheters was proximal (cephalad) migration noted. These latter 6 catheters required further manipulation. The total charges for the postprocedural chest radiographs were estimated at $21,735, or approximately $35 per film. It was concluded that the postprocedural films were not routinely required except at the discretion of the interventional radiologist. Although most cases were IJV punctures, Lucey et al. felt that the results applied to subclavian vein accesses as well, although some investigators feel that the subclavian route has a higher pneumothorax rate (60). Moreover, factors associated with migration of the catheter were identified and included obese patients or patients with pendulous breasts. Solutions suggested to minimize migration in such high-risk patients were to insert longer catheters and to use a medially placed tunnel onto the anterior chest wall.

Although somewhat controversial, the optimum location for the tip of central venous catheters is believed to be the SVC or high RA just central to the cavoatrial junction (37,62). One difficulty that has become apparent is the frequent migration of catheter tip location initially documented on supine intraprocedural views of the chest and subsequently on upright chest radiographs (63,64). Kowalski et al. studied 50 patients with supine maximum inspiratory chest radiographs on the angiography table immediately after catheter placement and delayed upright inspiratory chest radiographs obtained 2 to 24 hours after CVA (63). In the vast majority of cases (98%), there was cephalad migration of the catheter tip of 3.2 ± 1.8 cm (corrected for magnification). In one case, there was central migration of the catheter tip of 3.9 cm. Migration was a function of catheter type and was greatest with larger devices (12 Fr double-lumen port = 4.1 ± 2.1 cm vs. 10 Fr single-lumen port = 2.3 ± 1.6 cm). Based on their results, Kowalski et al. routinely place the catheter tip 3 to 4 cm more centrally than the desired tip position (63). The site of tunneling was also identified as important because the mobility of chest wall tissues may tether the catheter, causing catheter tip migration. Kowalski et al. noted a trend toward lower catheter malfunction and central vein thrombosis (3.4% vs. 18%) with the tip within the high RA than in the SVC, although the differences were not significant statistically (p = 0.2) (63). Nazarian and co-workers studied 146 different tunneled catheters from various sites (64). Catheter tip sites were numbered from 1 to 8: 1 = BCV-SVC junction and 8 = lower RA. Patient sex and weight, site of catheter entry, and size and type of catheters were correlated with change in position on follow-up radiographs. The study showed a significant change in catheter position with a mean difference of 1.5 positions. Migration was greatest for catheters in the subclavian veins, in female patients, and in obese patients. Nazarian et al. recommended using the IJV for access and using medially directed tunnels, especially in obese or female patients (64).

Too low a catheter position in the RA risks inducing cardiac arrhythmias, cardiac perforation, migration of the catheter into the IVC or hepatic veins, and RA thrombus (65–67). The U.S. Food and Drug Administration recommends avoiding RA tip positioning for all central vein catheters based on data derived from complications of central venous catheters, flexible or nonflexible (68). Unfortunately, the report did not differentiate between firmer temporary catheters and softer, silastic, tunneled catheters, which are more commonly inserted by interventionalists. The original descriptions of the Hickman and Broviac catheters referred to these catheters as "RA catheters" (69,70).

CONCLUSION

CVA techniques are crucial elements of the care of many patients in the modern era. The application of imaging and interventional tools to the insertion of the various venous access devices is safe, effective, and cost effective. Therefore, the domain of venous access is becoming increasingly a significant part of the interventional radiologist's workload. It is hoped that the reader has learned some of the valuable lessons available based on imaging so that venous access can be performed in the optimum manner.

REFERENCES

1. Alexander HR. Insertion technique for long-term venous access catheter: percutaneous subclavian vein cannulation. *Vascular access in the cancer patient.* Philadelphia: JB Lippincott, 1994.
2. Ryder MA. Peripherally inserted central venous catheters. *Nurs Clin North Am* 1993;28:937–971.
3. Seldinger SI. Catheter replacement of needle in percutaneous arteriography: a new technique. *Acta Radiol Diagn* 1982;39:368–376.
4. Noh HM, Kaufman JA, Fan CM, et al. Radiologic approach to central venous catheters: cost analysis. *Semin Intervent Radiol* 1998;15:335–340.
5. Ganz PA. The quality of life after breast cancer-solving the problem of lymphedema. *N Engl J Med* 1999; 340:383–385.
6. Polak JF, Anderson D, Hagspiel K, et al. Peripherally inserted central venous catheters: factors affecting patient satisfaction. *AJR* 1998;170:1609–1611.
7. Fraser JD, Anderson DN. Deep venous thrombosis: recent advances and optimal investigation with ultrasound. *Radiology* 1999;211:9–24.
8. Longley DG, Finlay DE, Letourneau JG. Sonography of the upper extremity and jugular veins. *AJR* 1993; 160:957–962.

9. Hightower DG, Gooding GAW. Sonographic evaluation of the normal response of subclavian vein to respiratory maneuvers. *Invest Radiol* 1985;20:517–520.

10. Wing V, Scheible W. Sonography of jugular vein thrombosis. *AJR* 1983;140:333–336.

11. Weissleder R, Elizondo G, Stark DD. Sonographic diagnosis of subclavian and internal jugular vein thrombosis. *J Ultrasound Med* 1987;6:577–587.

12. Valji K. Upper extremity veins and superior vena cava. *Vascular and interventional radiology.* In: Valji K, ed. Philadelphia: WB Saunders, 1999:316–336.

13. Benenati JF, Becker GJ, Mail JT, et al. Digital subtraction venography in central venous obstruction. *AJR* 1986;147:685–688.

14. Stanford W, Jolles H, Ell S, et al. Superior vena cava obstruction: a venographic classification. *AJR* 1987; 148:259–262.

15. Hahn ST, Pfammatter T, Cho KJ. Carbon dioxide gas a venous contrast agent to guide upper-arm insertion of central venous catheters. *Cardiovasc Intervent Radiol* 1995;18:146–149.

16. Kaufman JA, Geller SC, Waltman AC. Renal insufficiency: gadopentetate dimeglumine as a radiographic contrast agent during peripheral vascular interventional procedures. *Radiology* 1996;198:579–581.

17. Gorich VJ, Flentje M, Gückel F, et al. Computed tomographic imaging of collaterals in stenoses of large mediastinal veins. *ROFO* 1988:148:560–565

18. Goodwin JD, Wee WR. Contrast-related flow phenomena mimicking pathology on thoracic computed tomography. *J Comput Assist Tomogr* 1982;6:460–467.

19. Weinreb JC, Mootz A, Cohen JM. MRI evaluation of mediastinal and thoracic inlet venous obstruction. *AJR* 1986;146:679–684.

20. Finn JP, Zisk JHS, Edelman RR, et al. Central venous occlusion: MR angiography. *Radiology* 1993;187:245–251.

21. Rose SC, Gomes AS, Yoon HC. MR angiography for mapping potential central venous access sites in patients with advanced venous occlusive disease. *AJR* 1996;166:1181–1187.

22. Hartnell GG, Hughes LA, Finn JP, et al. Magnetic resonance angiography of the central chest veins. A new gold standard? *Chest* 1995;107:1053–1057.

23. Shinde TS, Lee VJ, Rofsky NM, et al. Three-dimensional gadolinium-enhanced MR venographic evaluation of central veins in the thorax: initial experience. *Radiology* 1999;213:555–560.

24. Lebowitz JA, Rofsky NM, Krinsky GA, et al. Gadolinium-enhanced body angiography with subtraction technique. *AJR* 1997;169:755–758.

25. Ballard JL, Smith LL. Surgical anatomy for vascular access procedures. In: Wilson SE, ed. *Vascular access: principles and practice,* 3rd ed. St. Louis: CV Mosby, 1996:19–27.

26. Armstrong PJ, Sutherland R, Scott DHT. The effect of position and different manoeuvers on internal jugular vein diameter size. *Acta Anaesthesiol Scand* 1994;38:229–231.

27. Aitken DR, Minton JP. The "pinch-off sign": a warning of impending problems with permanent subclavian catheters. *Am J Surg* 1984;148:633–636.

28. Namyslowski J, Patel NH. Central venous access: a new task for interventional radiologists. *Cardiovasc Intervent Radiol* 1999;22:355–368

29. Cimochowski GE, Worley E, Rutherford WE, et al. Superiority of the internal jugular over the subclavian access for temporary hemodialysis. *Nephron* 1990;54:154–161.

30. Vanherweghem JL, Yassine T, Goldman M, et al. Subclavian vein thrombosis: a frequent complication of subclavian vein cannulation for hemodialysis. *Clin Nephrol* 1986;26:235–238.

31. Clark DD, Albina JE, Chazan JA. Subclavian vein stenosis and thrombosis: a potential serious complication in chronic hemodialysis patients. *Am J Kidney Dis* 1990;15:265–268.

32. Barrett N, Spencer S, McIvor J, et al. Subclavian stenosis: a major complication of subclavian dialysis catheters. *Nephrol Dial Transplant* 1988;3:423–425.

33. Schwab SJ, Quarles LD, Middleton JP, et al. Hemodialysis-associated subclavian stenosis. *Kidney Int* 1988; 33:1156–1159.

34. Monreal M, Raventos A, Lerma R, et al. Pulmonary embolism in patients with upper-extremity DVT associated to venous central lines. A prospective study. *Thromb Haemost* 1994;72:548–550.

35. NKF-DOQI clinical practice guidelines for vascular access. National Kidney Foundation-dialysis outcomes quality initiative. *Am J Kidney Dis* 1997;30(suppl): 159–191.

36. Jaques PF, Campbell WE, Dumbleton S, et al. The first rib as a fluoroscopic marker for subclavian access. *J Vasc Intervent Radiol* 1995;6:619–622.

37. Mauro MA, Jaques PF. Radiologic placement of long-term central venous catheters: a review. *J Vasc Intervent Radiol* 1993;4:127–137.

38. Hovsepian DM, Bonn J, Eschelman DJ. Techniques for peripheral insertion of central venous catheters. *J Vasc Intervent Radiol* 1993;4:795–803.

39. Yeow KM, Kaufman JA, Rieumont MJ, et al. Axillary vein puncture over the second rib. *AJR* 1998;170:924–926.

40. Page AC, Evans RA, Kaczmarski R, et al. The insertion of chronic indwelling central venous catheters (Hickman lines) in interventional radiology suites. *Clin Radiol* 1990;42:105–109.

41. Silberzweig JE, Cooper JM, Podolak MJ, et al. Venography in the lordotic projection to facilitate central venous access. *J Vasc Intervent Radiol* 1996;7:439–440.

42. Shetty PC, Mody MK, Kastan DJ, et al. Outcome of 350 implanted chest ports placed by interventional radiologists. *J Vasc Intervent Radiol* 1997;8:991–995.

43. Aburahma AF, Sadler DL, Robinson PA. Axillary-subclavian vein thrombosis: changing patterns of etiology, diagnostic, and therapeutic modalities. *Am Surgeon* 1991;57:101–107.

44. Horattas MC, Wright DJ, Fenton AH, et al. Changing concepts of deep venous thrombosis of the upper extremity: report of a series and review of the literature. *Surgery* 1988;104:561–567.

45. Kerr TM, Lutter KS, Moeller DM, et al. Upper extremity venous thrombosis diagnosed by duplex scanning. *Am J Surg* 1990;160:202–206.

46. Axelsson CK, Efsen F. Phlebography in long-term catheterization of the subclavian vein: a retrospective study in patients with severe gastrointestinal disorders. *Scand J Gastroenterol* 1978;13:933–938.

47. Rose SC, Kinney TB, Bundens WP, et al. Importance of Doppler analysis of transmitted atrial waveforms prior

to placement of central venous access catheters. *J Vasc Intervent Radiol* 1998;9:927–934.

48. Silberzweig JE, Mitty HA. Central venous access: low internal jugular vein approach using imaging guidance. *AJR* 1998;170:1617–1620.
49. Trerotola SO, Johnson MS, Harris VJ, et al. Outcome of tunneled hemodialysis catheters placed via the right internal jugular vein by interventional radiologists. *Radiology* 1997;203:489–495.
50. Andrews JC, Marx MV, Williams DM, et al. The upper arm approach for placement of peripherally inserted central catheters for protracted venous access. *AJR* 1992;158:427–429.
51. Mansfield PF, Hohn DC, Fornage BD, et al. Complications and failures of subclavian-vein catheterization. *N Engl J Med* 1994;331:1735–1738.
52. Bambauer R, Inninger R, Pirrung KJ, et al. Complications and side effects associated with large-bore catheters in the subclavian and internal jugular veins. *Artif Organs* 1994;18:318–321.
53. Yerdel MA, Karayalcin K, Aras N, et al. Mechanical complications of subclavian vein catheterization. A prospective study. *Int Surg* 1991;76:18–22.
54. Denys BG, Uretsky BF, Reddy PS. Ultrasound-assisted cannulation of the internal jugular vein. A prospective comparison to the external landmark-guided technique. *Circulation* 1993;87:1557–1562.
55. Teichgräber, Benter T, Gebel M, et al. A sonographic guided technique for central venous access. *AJR* 1997;169:731–733.
56. Hawkins IF, Paige RM. Redirection of malpositioned central venous catheters. *AJR* 1983;140:393–394.
57. Spies JB, Berlin L. Complications of central venous catheter placement. *AJR* 1997;169:339–341.
58. Robertson AJ, Mauro MA, Jaques PF. Radiologic placement of Hickman catheters. *Radiology* 1989;170:1007–1009.
59. Muth CM, Shank ES. Gas embolism. *N Engl J Med* 2000;342:476–482.
60. Chang TC, Funaki B, Szymski GX. Are routine chest radiographs necessary after image-guided placement of internal jugular central venous access? *AJR* 1998;170:335–337.
61. Lucey B, Varghese JC, Haslam P, et al. Routine chest radiographs after central line insertion: mandatory postprocedural evaluation or unnecessary waste of resources? *Cardiovasc Intervent Radiol* 1999;22:381–384.
62. Openshaw KL, Vesely TM, Picus J. Interventional radiologic placement of Hohn central venous catheters: results and complications in 100 consecutive patients. *J Vasc Intervent Radiol* 1994;5:111–115.
63. Kowalski CM, Kaufman JA, Rivitz SM, et al. Migration of central venous catheters: implications for initial catheter tip positioning. *J Vasc Intervent Radiol* 1997;8:443–447.
64. Nazarian GW, Bjarnason H, Dietz CA, et al. Changes in tunneled catheter tip position when a patient is upright. *J Vasc Intervent Radiol* 1997;8:437–441.
65. Spotnitz WD, Dent JM, Mintz PD, et al. Removal of an infected right atrial mass in a patient with sickle cell disease. *Ann Thorac Surg* 1994;58:1762–1764.
66. Bivins MH, Callahan MJ. Position-dependent ventricular tachycardia related to a peripherally inserted central catheter. *Mayo Clin Proc* 2000;75:414–416.
67. Ellis PK, Kidney DD, Deutsch LS. Giant right atrial thrombus: a life-threatening complication of long-term central venous access catheters. *J Vasc Intervent Radiol* 1997;8:865–868.
68. Scott WL. Central venous catheters: an overview of Food and Drug Administration activities. *Surg Oncol Clin North Am* 1995;4:377–393.
69. Hickman RO, Buckner CD, Clift RA, et al. A modified right atrial catheter for access to the venous system in marrow transplant patients. *Surg Gynecol Obstet* 1979;148:871–875.
70. Broviac JW, Cole JJ, Scribner BH. A silicone rubber atrial catheter for prolonged parenteral alimentation. *Surg Gynecol Obstet* 1973;136:602–606.

Central Venous Access
Edited by Charles E. Ray, Jr.
Lippincott Williams & Wilkins, Philadelphia © 2001.

4

Preprocedural Assessment

Jan Namyslowski, MD

*University Hospital; Department of Radiology, Indiana University School of Medicine,
Indianapolis, Indiana 46202-5253*

Even though central venous catheter placement appears a relatively simple and straightforward procedure, paying attention to the details is necessary to prevent potentially dangerous complications. An example of such a complication is illustrated in Figs. 4.1 to 4.3. In this patient, an unrecognized through-and-through internal jugular vein (IJV) puncture resulted in a subclavian artery transection and extravascular catheter placement into the chest cavity. This necessitated emergency surgery with placement of an interposition subclavian artery graft and ligation of the IJV. If the anatomic relationship of the adjacent IJV and subclavian artery had been recognized before the procedure, the complication would have been far less likely to occur.

DEVICE SELECTION

Device selection influences the extent to which the preprocedural patient assessment needs to be performed. Therefore, albeit somewhat counterintuitive, one should first thoroughly assess the infusion requirements demanding device placement in the first place. Device selection depends on the composition of infusates, the frequency of administration, and duration of treatment. Hyperosmolar solutions should only be delivered into large central veins, such as the superior vena cava or inferior vena cava (IVC). Other issues to be considered include venous anatomic variations; a history of prior intervention or surgery at the planned access site; pathologic processes affecting the insertion point and pertinent venous network; cost; and physician or patient preference (1).

Although tunneled devices and ports generally are offered for long-term and occasionally for intermediate-term use, one should bear in mind that nontunneled devices also may function successfully for a period of several weeks. Examples include centrally placed Hohn silastic catheters (Bard Access Systems, Salt Lake City, UT, U.S.A.) and percutaneously inserted central catheters (PICCs); these devices have reported implantation periods of up to 70 to 85 days and 28 to 73 days, respectively (2–5). PICCs have been used successfully in the administration of total parenteral nutrition (TPN) (6–8), thus obviating the need for a tunneled device; in contrast, ports should not be used for TPN administration because of an increased infection rate (9).

Device selection dictates the extent of patient workup. A coagulation screen is necessary when planning the insertion of a tunneled catheter or a subcutaneous port. To the contrary, a coagulopathy should not be viewed as a contraindication to placement of short-term nontunneled lines, provided the access is image guided. The same guidelines may be used for patients who are thrombocytopenic. The indications, advantages, and disadvantages of basic types of devices are reviewed and summarized in Table 4.1.

PREPROCEDURAL EVALUATION

Once the most optimal device has been selected, patient assessment should begin. As indicated above, its extent will be dictated primarily by the choice of a nontunneled or a tunneled device, the latter requiring a much more elaborate preprocedure evaluation. The

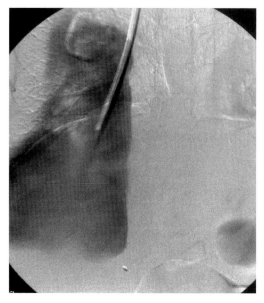

FIG. 4.1. An abnormal course of tunneled dialysis catheter was noted on the postplacement chest radiograph. The catheter placement was uneventful, according to the operator. Contrast injection demonstrates the catheter to be in the pleural cavity.

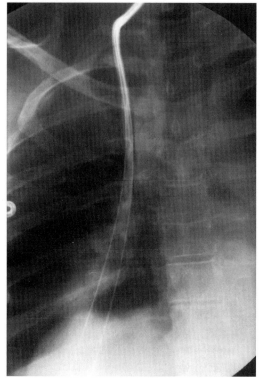

FIG. 4.2. In the same patient shown in Fig. 4.1, two guidewires were inserted to facilitate a pullback injection without losing access.

main limiting factor in the tunneled device (ports included) group is the presence of uncorrectable coagulopathy and bacteremia. At my institution, the minimum requirements are systemic infection-free state or a set of two negative blood cultures in a patient previously shown to have been bacteremic, as well as platelet count and international normalized ratio (INR) of greater than or equal to 50,000/mm³ and 1.5 units, respectively. If necessary, corrective measures are taken and include the administration of fresh frozen plasma at 15 mL/kg and a transfusion of platelets; a 10,000/mm³ increase in the platelet count typically follows a transfusion of 1 unit of platelets (10). On the other hand, a short-term nontunneled IJV central venous catheter or a PICC may be placed with little additional risk in patients who are coagulopathic or in the setting of an active infection.

The patient's history of prior venous access is an important next consideration. For example, it is well known that prior, especially repetitive,

cannulation of the subclavian vein frequently causes venous stenosis or occlusion (11–14). An attempt to place a PICC via the ipsilateral upper extremity venous system may be a time-consuming exercise in futility. For this reason, physical examination should be a mandatory part of preprocedural workup. As it pertains to potential iatrogenic effects of prior catheterization, physical examination may reveal an abundant superficial collateral network, thus offering a clue to the possibility of an underlying central venous occlusion. In the presence of a previously documented vascular occlusion and development of a collateral network, one should consider the potential impact of using one of the collateral vessels as an access route on the venous drainage from the affected area. If a single, large collateral vessel is present, its potential device-related thrombosis might significantly impair venous outflow. The diminished ability

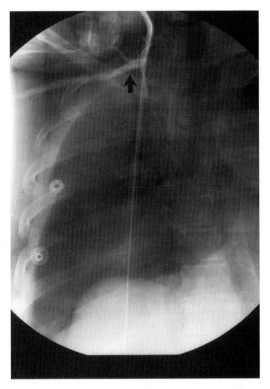

FIG. 4.3. In the same patient as shown in Figs. 4.1 and 4.2, a pullback injection demonstrates contrast material opacifying the partly transected right subclavian artery (*arrow*).

of an already compromised system to further develop collateral veins may result in significant symptomatology for the patient.

Physical examination also should include an assessment of the skin at the venous entry site. Postradiation changes, active skin infection, tracheostomy, skin neoplasms, and other dermatologic disorders may all dictate choosing a different vascular entry site. A history of prior venous intervention, such as placement of a stent bridging the brachiocephalic and subclavian veins, is important to know because it may potentially preclude an ipsilateral IJV access, unless a catheter is placed through the interstices of the previously placed stent. A history of prior surgery, for example a radical neck dissection (RND), is also important because the IJV is removed in the process; even modified RND may result in IJV removal (15). One should also be aware of prior caval filter place-

ment and the existence of any *in situ* venous access devices, because the needles, catheters, or wires used during venous access device placement may perforate or become entangled with the devices already in place. (16, 17)

Image-guided central venous device placement rarely requires an injection of iodinated contrast material. PICC placement under venographic guidance and the potential need to image central veins in a setting of unsuspected central venous occlusion may constitute exceptions. Therefore, the patient's renal function and any allergies, including allergies to iodinated contrast agents, should be investigated by the operator before the procedure. Because contrast agent may be used in any patient, including those in whom ultrasonographic guidance is anticipated, obtaining a preprocedure history of renal function and allergies is mandatory.

In most complex cases involving known central venous occlusions, strong consideration should be given to preprocedural imaging of the central veins, which may allow for a precise venous mapping and planning of safe and effective access site. Although duplex Doppler ultrasonography is typically the least expensive and most readily available method by which to interrogate the veins (Figs. 4.4 and 4.5), it can only assess the most central veins (brachiocephalic veins and superior vena cava) by secondary findings. The most accurate visualization of all the central veins is typically achieved with magnetic resonance venography, although drawbacks such as cost and availability may severely limit its utility (Fig. 4.6).

Antibiotic prophylaxis in central venous access is somewhat controversial, and the literature on the subject is inconsistent. There are no conclusive data to support antibiotic prophylaxis in nontunneled device placement; at least two randomized trials demonstrate no benefit in reducing the incidence of subsequent infections (18,19). Similarly, two reports show no benefit to antibiotic prophylaxis in patients undergoing tunneled dialysis catheter placement (20,21). Conversely, Simpson et al. (22) demonstrated a low infection rate in patients receiving subcutaneous ports when antibiotic prophylaxis was given. For these reasons, the current antibiotic

TABLE 4.1. *Relative characteristics and merits of selected devices*

Temporary catheters	PICC	Tunneled external catheters	Implanted ports
Indications			
Short-term/intermediate use	Short-term/intermediate use	Long-term continuous (intermittent) use	Long-term intermittent (continuous) use
Continuous/intermittent use	Continuous/intermittent use	Short-/long-term high-low applications	
High-flow applications			
Advantages			
Rapid, inexpensive access to central venous system	Eliminates repetitive needle sticks	Higher flow rates	Lower infection rate
	Allows outpatient therapy	No needle sticks	Lower maintenance
		Lower cost	Fewer activity limitations
Disadvantages			
Limited duration of use	Limited duration of use—expense in placement if done in IR suite	Higher infection rate	Repetitive needle sticks
Placement-related complications with landmark technique		Daily maintenance	Initial expense in placement
Infection rate	Limited in high-volume applications	More activity limitations	
		Cosmetic concerns	
	Cosmetic concerns and activity limitations		

PICC, peripherally inserted central catheter; IR, interventional radiology.
Adapted from Namyslowski J, Patel NH. Central venous access: a new task for interventional radiologists.
Cardiovasc Intervent Radiol 1999;22:355–368.

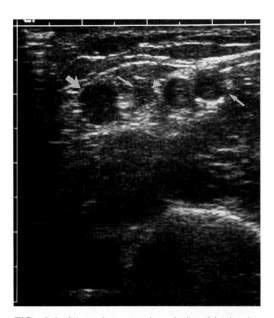

FIG. 4.4. Normal anatomic relationship in the arm is demonstrated. Basilic vein (*large arrow*) is seen medially; paired brachial veins (*small arrows*) are immediately adjacent to the brachial artery (*arrowhead*).

prophylaxis in central venous access at the author's institution is limited to subcutaneous port placement. We administer an intravenous (IV) antistaphylococcal agent, typically 1 g of cefazolin, within 1 hour prior to the procedure. In cases of allergy to cephalosporins or penicillins, we use levofloxacin 500 mg IV, again in a one-time preprocedural dose.

An assessment of the patient's medication list is mandatory prior to placing a venous access device. In addition to gaining valuable information on pertinent histories such as treatment of vascular disease or hypertension, the presence of certain specific drugs should be sought. In particular, diabetic patients who are either on oral hypoglycemic medications or insulin should have their medications adjusted in anticipation of undergoing any procedure. In particular, if the patient is taking metformin (Glucophage, Bristol Myers Squibb, Princeton, NJ, U.S.A.), there is the possibility of inducing a metabolic acidosis or worsening renal insufficiency once the patient is exposed to IV iodi-

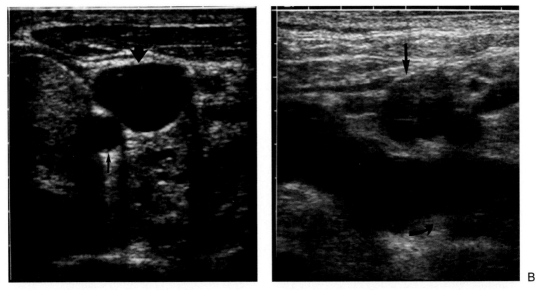

FIG. 4.5. Arterial/venous relationships in the supraclavicular area. Although the image **(A)** demonstrates the internal jugular vein (*large arrow*) and common carotid artery (*small arrow*) immediately posterior and medial to the vein, one should be aware that, especially closer to the clavicle **(B)**, the subclavian artery (*curved arrow*) may be located immediately posterior and transversely, relative to the internal jugular vein (*straight arrow*). Unless recognized, an inadvertent arterial entry may occur, as illustrated in Figs. 4.1 to 4.3.

nated contrast material. Although protocols vary, it is generally recommended that patients discontinue use of metformin the morning of their procedure, and do not resume the medication until at least 48 hours following the procedure. Some institutions require the patient to have

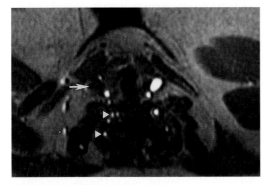

FIG. 4.6. Breath-hold gradient-echo magnetic resonance image demonstrating right internal jugular vein obstruction (*arrow*) with collateral flow via the posterior vertebral collateral system (*arrowheads*).

drawn a repeat serum creatinine level, and reinitiate the metformin only after the creatinine level has been shown to be the same both before and after the procedure.

Insulin doses are also typically adjusted before a procedure. The reason for such adjustments is that patients are typically denied food for at least 12 hours prior to their procedure. If patients were to take their entire insulin dose without eating, they would become severely hypoglycemic during the procedure. Many interventionalists have patients decrease their morning insulin dose by half, whereas others may completely discontinue the short-acting regular insulin but still have the patient take the longer acting derivatives. The advantage of drawing routine intraprocedural blood glucose levels has not been completely evaluated.

CHOICE OF VENOUS ENTRY SITE

Once the patient evaluation has been completed, ultrasonographic examination of the venous entry site should be performed. This may reveal an unsuspected venous thrombosis and allows the assessment of pertinent venous anatomy (Figs. 4.5 and 4.6). For example, the absence of the basilic vein may be identified or, in case of IJV access, its relationship to the common carotid artery or presence of the subclavian artery immediately posterior to the IJV at the venous entry site may be shown. The distinction between the veins and arteries is generally simple, with veins compressing readily under the ultrasonographic probe, although occasionally the brachial artery compresses as easily as the accompanying brachial vein; in cases of doubt, Doppler flow assessment allows for correct identification of the vein.

The right IJV is the preferred venous entry site for all nontunneled and tunneled devices, including ports and excluding PICCs, which are inserted via peripheral upper extremity veins. The reason for IJV preference is because the more traditional approach, the subclavian vein (SCV), is associated with a high incidence of venous stenosis and occlusion (11–14). Although this may be of no consequence in otherwise healthy patients, it does become a significant problem in the hemodialysis population. If the right IJV is occluded, the left IJV is the recommended access vein. The commonly held belief that the left-sided catheters do not fare well is likely related to the fact that the data available on such devices often are based on the catheter tip being located much further cephalad, frequently at the junction of the brachiocephalic veins, such that the device tip is directed toward the venous wall. We have shown that there is not a significant difference in the flow rates between the left- and right-sided IJV dialysis catheters as long as the catheter tip is positioned at least at the cavoatrial junction (23). If both IJVs are occluded, then the external jugular vein (EJV) is a viable option to consider. However, the device often kinks when the EJV is used as an entry for tunneled catheter placement. On the other hand, provided that the superior vena cava can be accessed, the EJV is a perfectly acceptable route for a nontunneled catheter.

If both the IJVs and EJVs are occluded, a decision has to be made whether or not to continue to attempt to gain access above the diaphragm. Other than PICC placement, which may or may not be appropriate given the indication for device placement, the only remaining possible venous access site is the SCV. A more lateral approach to the SCV entry, such as over the lateral aspect of the first or second rib, has been described and might be a viable option in certain patients (24,25). Depending on the appropriateness of SCV placement, the next option would be to place a device directly into the IVC via a translumbar approach (26). In rare circumstances, a transhepatic route (27) may be considered, although fewer data are available on the performance of these lines, and their maintenance and function are generally more problematic. The choice of alternate access sites is discussed in detail in Chapter 12.

Finally, patients with end-stage renal disease require special mention, especially as it pertains to PICC placement. According to the Dialysis Outcome Quality Initiative recommendations (28), peripheral veins should be preserved in such patients for the purpose of a future arteriovenous dialysis access creation. We have developed a technique of placement of tunneled small-bore central catheters, placed via the IJV, to avoid the use of peripheral veins (29). We are presently using serum creatinine values of 3.0 or greater as an indication to place such a device in lieu of PICC placement. Although somewhat arbitrary, this does underscore the need to establish one's own hospital policy in this regard by consulting with the nephrologists and transplant surgeons.

SUMMARY

Careful attention to a number of important issues in preprocedural assessment, as outlined in this chapter, allows placement of the most appropriate device in a most effective way, thus creating a reliable, efficient, and successful service.

REFERENCES

1. Namyslowski J, Patel NH. Central venous access: a new task for interventional radiologists. *Cardiovasc Intervent Radiol* 1999;22:355–368.

2. Openshaw Kl, Picus D, Hicks ME, et al. Interventional radiologic placement of Hohn central venous catheters: results and complications in 100 consecutive patients. *JVIR* 1994;5:111–115.
3. Raad I, Davis S, Becker M, et al. Low infection rate and long durability of nontunneled silastic catheters. A safe and cost-effective alternative for long-term venous access. *Arch Intern Med* 1993;153:1791–1796.
4. Cardella JF, Fox PS, Lawler JB. Interventional radiologic placement of peripherally inserted central catheters. *JVIR* 1993;4:653–660.
5. Cardella JF, Cardella K, Bacci N, et al. Cumulative experience with 1,273 peripherally inserted central catheters at a single institution. *JVIR* 1996;7:5–13.
6. Yeung CY, Lee HC, Huang FY, et al. Sepsis during total parenteral nutrition: exploration of risk factors and determination of the effectiveness of peripherally inserted central venous catheters. *Pediatr Infect Dis J* 1998; 17:135–142.
7. Alhimyary A, Fernandez C, Picard M, et al. Safety and efficacy of total parenteral nutrition delivered via a peripherally inserted central venous catheter. *Nutr Clin Pract* 1996;11:199–203.
8. Loughran SC, Borzatta M. Peripherally inserted catheters: a report of 2506 catheter days. *J Parenter Enter Nutr* 1995;19:133–136.
9. Pearson ML. Guideline for prevention of intravascular device-related infections. *Infect Control Hosp Epidemiol* 1996;17:438–473.
10. Namyslowski, J, Trerotola SO. Management of hypotension and hemorrhage: the principles of prevention, diagnosis and therapy. In: Murphy TP, Benenati JF, Kaufman JA, eds. *Patient care in interventional radiology.* Fairfax, VA: Society of Cardiovascular and Interventional Radiology, 1999:55–65.
11. Cimochowski GE, Worley E, Rutherford WE, et al. Superiority of the internal jugular over the subclavian access for temporary hemodialysis. *Nephron* 1990;54:154–161.
12. Schillinger F, Schillinger D, Montagnac R, et al. Central venous stenosis in hemodialysis: comparative angiographic study of subclavian and internal jugular access. *Nephrologie* 1994;15:129–131.
13. Beenen L, van Leusen R, Deenik B, et al. The incidence of subclavian vein stenosis using silicone catheters for hemodialysis. *Artif Organs* 1994;18:289–292.
14. Macdonald S, Watt AJB, Edwards RD, et al. Comparison of the internal jugular and subclavian venous routes in radiographically placed tunneled venous access lines. *Cardiovasc Intervent Radiol* 1998;21(suppl 1):81.
15. Rush BF. Tumors of the head and neck. In: Schwartz SI, Shires GT, Spencer FC, eds. *Principles of surgery,* 5th ed. New York: McGraw-Hill, 1989:581–626.
16. Kaufman JA, Thomas JW, Geller SC, et al. Guide-wire entrapment by inferior vena cava filters: in vitro evaluation. *Radiology* 1996;198:71–76.
17. Loesberg A, Taylor FC, Awh MH. Dislodgement of inferior vena caval filters during "blind" insertion of central venous catheters. *AJR* 1993;161:637–638.
18. Ranson MR, Oppenheim BA, Jackson A, et al. Double-blind placebo controlled study of vancomycin prophylaxis for central venous catheter insertion in cancer patients. *J Hosp Infect* 1990;15:95–102.
19. McKee R, Dunsmuir R, Whitby M, et al. Does antibiotic prophylaxis at the time of catheter insertion reduce the incidence of catheter-related sepsis in intravenous nutrition? *J Hosp Infect* 1985;6:419–425.
20. Trerotola SO, Johnson MS, Harris VJ, et al. Outcome of tunneled hemodialysis catheters placed via the right IJV by interventional radiologists. *Radiology* 1997; 203:489–495.
21. Lund GB, Trerotola SO, Scheel PF, et al. Outcome of tunneled hemodialysis catheters placed by radiologists. *Radiology* 1996;198:467–472.
22. Simpson KR, Hovsepian DM, Picus D. Interventional radiologic placement of chest wall ports: results and complications in 161 consecutive placements. *JVIR* 1997;8:189–195.
23. Namyslowski J, Trerotola SO, McKusky M, et al. Retrospective analysis of blood flow rates via tunneled right and left internal jugular vein dialysis catheters. *Cardiovasc Intervent Radiol* 1999;22(suppl 2):91.
24. Fan CM. Tunneled catheters. *Semin Intervent Radiol* 1998;15:273–286.
25. Jaques P, Campbell WE, Dumbleton S, et al. The first rib as a fluoroscopic marker for subclavian vein access. *JVIR* 1995;6:619–622.
26. Kenney PR, Dorfman GS, Denny DF. Percutaneous inferior vena cava cannulation for long-term parenteral access. *Surgery* 1985;97:602–605.
27. Crummy AB, Carlson P, McDermott JC, et al. Percutaneous transhepatic placement of a Hickman catheter. *AJR* 1989;153:1317–1318.
28. NKF-DOQI clinical practice guidelines for vascular access. National Kidney Foundation-dialysis outcomes quality initiative. *Am J Kidney Dis* 1997;30 (suppl): 150–191.
29. Sasadeusz KJ, Trerotola SO, Shah H, et al. Tunneled jugular small-bore central catheters as an alternative to peripherally inserted central catheters for intermediate-term venous access in patients with hemodialysis and chronic renal insufficiency. *Radiology* 1999;213: 303–306.

Central Venous Access
Edited by Charles E. Ray, Jr.
Lippincott Williams & Wilkins, Philadelphia © 2001.

5

Short- and Intermediate-Term Central Venous Catheters

Jan Namyslowski, MD and *Charles E. Ray, Jr., MD

*University Hospital; Department of Radiology, Indiana University School of Medicine,
Indianapolis, Indiana 46202-5253; *Denver Health Medical Center;
University of Colorado Health Sciences Center, Denver, Colorado 80204*

In the late 1920s, Forssman performed central venous catheterization on himself by passing "a well oiled 4F ureteric catheter up to the heart" from an antecubital access. He then obtained a chest radiograph on himself, confirming the central venous position of the catheter; this was perhaps the first recorded case of radiologic confirmation of central venous catheter (CVC) position (1). This accomplishment, together with the first human central venous catheterization in 1905 by Bleichroder, set the stage for the development and refinement of this important procedure. Keeri-Szanto (2) popularized the infraclavicular subclavian vein approach in a study using cadavers in 1956; the ease of placement and lack of anatomically evident complications proved the route to be clinically useful. However, increasing frequency of central venous access by this route was accompanied by a high complication rate, and descriptions of the supraclavicular and internal jugular vein approaches soon followed (1,3). Finally, in complicated patients, such as those with previous line-related venous thromboses, alternative access routes (inferior vena cava, transhepatic) were developed in the 1980s (4–6).

CATHETER TYPES AND CLINICAL INDICATIONS

In most patients admitted to the hospital, venous access is accomplished through the use of peripheral intravenous catheters (IVs). Drawbacks to the use of IVs, however, include the inability to draw blood samples from them, the requirement that the insertion site be changed every few days to decrease the risk of phlebitis, the lack of palpable or visible peripheral veins in certain patients, and potential lack of resources (e.g., a dedicated IV team) to place or care for the IV. Certain fluids, such as concentrated antibiotics or chemotherapy agents, also may sclerose smaller peripheral veins, rendering them unavailable for future venipunctures; such fluids may be more safely given via a central vein. In addition, certain infusion therapies (e.g., total parenteral nutrition) must be given directly into the central venous system, because of the composition of the infusate. Finally, in patients who are acutely ill, large volumes of fluid may be required, and measurement of central venous pressures may be helpful in determining the best course of care for the patient. All of these ends are best accomplished using CVCs.

In addition to the above reasons used for placement of a CVC in patients requiring hospitalization, many outpatients who receive IV therapy also may benefit from some form of CVC placement. Particularly in patients who will receive only a short course of outpatient IV therapy, permanent devices (e.g., tunneled catheters and ports) are not required and, indeed, add significantly to the cost of therapy.

TABLE 5.1. *General categories of central venous catheters*

Duration of therapy		
Short (<2 wk)	Intermediate (2 wk to 2 mo)	Long (>2 mo)
Peripheral IV catheters Temporary dialysis catheters Temporary central PVC catheters Monitoring central catheters	PICCs Temporary central silicone catheters	Tunneled catheters Implantable devices

IV, intravenous; PICC, peripherally inserted central catheter; PVC, polyvinyl chloride

The type of device chosen for central venous access depends in large part on the duration of therapy (Table 5.1). In this chapter, we focus on short-term and intermediate-term CVCs via a central approach; peripherally inserted central catheters (PICCs), which represent a form of intermediate-term CVCs via a peripheral approach, are discussed in Chapter 9. Temporary dialysis catheters are also discussed in Chapter 8, which addresses hemodialysis catheters.

The clinical indications for placement of a CVC vary widely from institution to institution. In some patients, the decision is easily made; patients who are hemodynamically unstable, for instance, and who require large volumes of fluid or constant central venous pressure monitoring should all receive a CVC. At the other end of the spectrum lie patients in whom CVC placement is largely a comfort issue, for example, patients who require frequent blood draws, or those with diminutive peripheral veins in whom venipunctures are difficult and uncomfortable. With the added safety margin of placing a CVC under imaging guidance (discussed later), and with the increased reliance on outpatient management, the indications for CVC placement have broadened significantly.

As outlined in Table 5.1, most of the patients in whom CVC placement is anticipated to be under 2 weeks' duration would benefit from a short-term CVC. These catheters, largely made of polyurethane, may be used for up to 2 weeks at a time without being replaced. Additionally, if the patient requires central venous access for longer than 2 weeks, the catheter may be exchanged over a wire using the same site for an-

other 2 weeks. The major benefit of such temporary polyurethane catheters is cost savings; when compared with intermediate-term silicone-based catheters, the cost savings is typically 50% or greater. Drawbacks to this category of catheters include the short duration of time the catheters may dwell in place; one catheter change using the over-a-wire technique more than negates the cost savings, especially when technical and physician fees are included. In addition, many home health-care agencies do not provide care for polyurethane-based catheters on an outpatient setting. For these reasons, it might prove advantageous to place an intermediate-term catheter initially in a patient in whom outpatient care is anticipated.

In terms of CVCs, the length of "intermediate duration" is debatable. In the dialysis population, the Dialysis Outcome Quality Initiative (7) recommends that a tunneled catheter be placed if the duration of catheterization is to exceed 3 weeks. In the nondialysis population, intermediate-term, nontunneled CVCs have been placed routinely for durations up to 85 days (8,9). Generally speaking, the clinical indications for placement of a central intermediate-term catheter (e.g., Hohn catheter, Bard Access Systems, Salt Lake City, UT, U.S.A.) include any patient who requires the CVC for 2 weeks to 2 months. Such patients may include individuals undergoing a short course of chemotherapy, or those in whom chemotherapy will be given intermittently and in whom an indwelling CVC would prove disadvantageous or undesirable. A second group of patients who may benefit from such an intermediate-term device would be individuals requiring long-term IV antibiotic therapy, such as patients with bacterial endocarditis or osteomyelitis. The benefit of intermediate-term CVC clearly lies in the fact that the devices may dwell in the patient for up to 2 months at a time; catheter exchange over a wire, assuming that the skin entry site appears normal, also may be performed. Drawbacks to such devices include cost and the need for daily or every-other-day care of the catheter (dressing changes and flushes).

CATHETER MATERIALS AND CHARACTERISTICS

Most temporary CVCs are made of polyurethane, the advantage of which is excellent tensile strength; this allows for a catheter with a large inner lumen while maintaining a small outer diameter. Polyurethanes are stiff enough to allow percutaneous insertion without an introducer sheath, yet they soften in response to body temperature. In some devices, the catheter tip is fashioned from a silicone elastomer in order to soften it further, potentially aiding in preventing possible endothelial damage. Polyurethanes may be bonded with a variety of substances. A cationic surfactant may be applied, allowing bonding of medications with the catheter surface (e.g., anionic antibiotics). Silver sulfadiazine and chlorhexidine also may be bonded to polyurethane, which may reduce the rate of bacterial colonization and catheter-related bacteremia.

Intermediate-term devices are typically made of silicone or silicone-based materials. PICCs are also typically fashioned from silicone, but some devices are made of polyurethane in an attempt to increase the "pushability" of the catheter. The most common type of central intermediate-term catheter is a silicone-based catheter, generally ranging in diameter from 5 to 7 French. Catheters may possess either single or double lumens, and may be purchased with or without a tissue ingrowth cuff on the catheter shaft. Because most catheters are made of silicone, they have poor inherent pushability. That characteristic, coupled with the fact that most catheters are blunt tipped and are inserted over a 0.025-inch diameter wire, can make place-

ment difficult. For these reasons, using a peel-away sheath may prove helpful when placing such catheters.

PATIENT PREPARATION

The standard preprocedural assessment prior to placement of a central venous device is listed in Table 5.2 (10–13). Abnormal laboratory values should not be considered an absolute contraindication to placement of a temporary device, but may suggest placement of one type of catheter over another. For instance, in a patient with an uncorrectable coagulopathy, an intermediate-term catheter should be placed rather than an implantable or tunneled device to decrease the risk of uncontrollable bleeding. The presence of bacteremia should also dissuade an operator from placing a tunneled or implantable device, which would place the permanent device at risk for secondary infection. In such instances, a short- or intermediate-term catheter may prove to be the best option until the patient's bacteremia resolves.

Patients with thrombocytopenia also may safely undergo catheter placement (14), although strict adherence to imaging-guided techniques is mandatory to prevent puncture of adjacent vital structures (e.g., arteries, pleura). Additionally, in patients with an uncorrectable coagulopathy or

TABLE 5.2. *Preprocedural patient assessment*

Prior catheterization history
Prior surgical history in the head, neck and chest area
Known venous anomalies
Prior trauma at the insertion site
Unilateral lung pathology
Mediastinal pathology
Laboratory studies (hematocrit, platelet count, INR)

INR, international normalized ratio.
Adapted from Namyslowski J. Temporary acute care central venous access devices. *Semin Intervent Radiol* 1998;15:253–258; with permission.
Data from Andris DA, Krzywda EA. Central venous access. Clinical practice issues. *Nurs Clin North Am* 1997;32:719–740; Whitman ED. Complications associated with the use of central venous access devices. *Curr Probl Surg* 1996;33:312–369; and Mansfield PF, Hohn DC, Fornage BD, et al. Complications and failures of subclavian-vein catheterization. *N Engl J Med* 1994;331:1735–1738.

TABLE 5.3. *Indications for image-guided placement of temporary central venous catheter*

Uncorrectable coagulopathy
Prior history of a difficult access or known stenoses or occlusions
Body mass index of >30 or <20
Certain clinical study protocol requirements

Adapted from Namyslowski J. Temporary acute care central venous access devices. *Semin Intervent Radiol* 1998;15:253–258; with permission.

thrombocytopenia, using lidocaine with epinephrine as the local anesthetic may aid in preventing bleeding from the skin vessels.

The indications for placement of a temporary catheter in the interventional radiology (IR) suite, as opposed to bedside placement, vary from institution to institution. The availability of housestaff or PICC nurses, as well as the availability of the IR service, largely determines when a line is placed by IR. Certain indications are generally more widely accepted; these indications for IR-placed CVCs are presented in Table 5.3. Of note, it is not uncommon, in the authors' experience, to place short- or intermediate-term catheters at the bedside using ultrasonographic guidance. This technique, while more time consuming for the IR staff, is often the most efficient method to place devices in certain patient populations (e.g., intensive care unit patients who require close monitoring). Additionally, bedside placement is very helpful if the IR suite is busy with cases strictly requiring fluoroscopy; the IR suite can then remain available for patients who absolutely require the equipment.

PLACEMENT TECHNIQUES AND RELATED ISSUES

Anatomic landmark techniques have been used for many years, and the reported surgical success rates for CVC placement using such techniques range from 95% to 100% (15). There is an ever-growing body of evidence indicating that image-guided central venous access is as successful and is associated with a lower complication rate when compared with placement using the anatomic landmark technique (8,10,13,16). Denys et al. found the internal jugular vein located outside the path predicted by the anatomic landmarks in over 5% of patients (17). Care must be taken when reviewing the literature regarding the degree of guidance offered by the imaging studies. For instance, one study concluded that ultrasonographic guidance offered no benefit in subclavian vein access guidance. In this study, however, the patients assigned to the "ultrasound-guided" group had their subclavian vein marked on the skin, after which the needle puncture occurred without real-time sonographic guidance (12). Data from several studies comparing the landmark and sonographic techniques are compiled in Tables 5.4 and 5.5 (16, 18–22). The published guidelines for image-guided central venous access are reflected in the Society of Cardiovascular and Interventional Radiology (SCVIR) Guidelines for Central Venous Access (23).

There is a paucity of studies assessing catheters placed in the common femoral vein (CFV). Trottier et al. (24) reported a 25% incidence of lower extremity deep venous thrombosis in patients with venous catheters inserted via CFV

TABLE 5.4. *Results of landmark technique*

Investigator	Access site	Overall success (success at first attempt)	Time (mean seconds)	Complications
Agee (21)	IJV	90%–95% (?)	?	2%
Ledgerwood (19)	SCV	90%–95% (?)	?	2%–5%
Denys (20)	IJV	88.1% (38%)	44.5	8.3%
Teichgraber (16)	IJV	52% (52%)	51.4	12%
Sznajder (22)	IJV, EJV, SCV	85.4% (?)	?	5.8%–11%
Farrell (18)	IJV	82% (35.9%)	?	7.7%

IJV, internal jugular vein; SCV, subclavian vein; EJV, external jugular vein.
Adapted from Namyslowski J. Temporary acute care central venous access devices. *Semin Intervent Radiol* 1998;15:253–258; with permission.

TABLE 5.5. *Results of ultrasonographically-guided techniques*

Investigator	Access site	Overall success (success at first attempt)	Time (mean seconds)	Complications
Denys (20)	IJV	100% (78%)	9.8	1.7%
Teichgraber (16)	IJV	96% (96%)	15.2	0%
Farrell (18)	IJV	96.7% (83.3%)	?	0%

IJV, internal jugular vein.
Adapted from Namyslowski J. Temporary acute care central venous access devices. *Semin Intervent Radiol* 1998;15:253–258; with permission.

access, compared with none in the group of subclavian/internal jugular vein insertions. This study, however, was limited by the small number of patients (n = 45) and the nondiagnostic quality of a significant percentage (29%) of the lower extremity ultrasonography examinations. The evidence in regard to presumably increased infection rate at this insertion site suffers from similar limitations. One investigator identified a 34% colonization rate at the femoral insertion site as opposed to 15% at the subclavian insertion site (25). In this study, however, the femoral catheters remained *in situ* for a longer period of time, and when an adjustment for this variable was made there was no significant difference between the femoral and internal/external jugular insertion sites; the subclavian catheters demonstrated a significantly lower colonization rate. In a third study, a higher rate of colonization was noted for femoral catheters (47%) when compared with internal jugular (22%) and subclavian (10%) vein catheters (26). This study, however, was also limited by the relatively low number of femoral catheters placed (n = 15). The Guideline for Prevention of Intravascular Device-Related Infections, published in 1996, identified a higher number of lumens and the insertion site as two of the risk factors for catheter-related infections (27). The subclavian vein insertion site demonstrated the lowest infection rate compared with the internal jugular and common femoral vein sites; the latter two sites were not distinguished by different rates (27).

COMPLICATIONS

Immediate complications of imaging-guided CVC placement are exceedingly rare. The incidence of pneumothorax, especially when a

jugular vein approach is used, is 1% or less; clinically significant pneumothoraces (i.e., those requiring chest tube placement) are nearly negligible (8,14,20,28). Similarly, the arterial puncture rate is extremely low and usually inconsequential, especially when a 21-gauge needle is used for the initial access.

Infectious complications represent the most common delayed complication noted with short- or intermediate-term CVCs. Due to the short duration of dwell time for short-term devices, infections are especially rare and typically treated by simply removing the catheter. In the published experience with intermediate-term catheters, a catheter infection rate of 0.9 to 1.1/1,000 catheter-days has been noted; a subclavian vein thrombosis rate of 3% also was found (8,9). Of interest, there is a high disparity between the rate of catheter removal for a suspected infection (25%) and the rate of catheter-related bacteremia as demonstrated by quantitative catheter cultures (3%) (9). This underscores the need for a thorough and adequate diagnosis of catheter-related infection before a catheter is removed.

CONCLUSIONS

Given the body of literature in support of image-guided central venous access, an important question to be answered is whether the interventional radiologist should be the sole provider of temporary catheter placement service. Although there are substantial cost savings when comparing radiologic versus surgical placement of long-term devices, there clearly is an increased cost when comparing radiologic placement of temporary CVCs versus those placed at the bedside. Additionally, although there is no doubt that ultrasonographically guided internal jugular vein access is associated with a lower complication rate and a higher success rate when compared with the landmark technique (16,18–22), the availability of this service, particularly in emergency situations, is limited at best. Therefore, we believe the landmark-guided temporary central venous access should continue to be taught and practiced, with image-guided placement reserved for the indications listed in Table 5.3. In summary, the temporary and intermediate duration central venous catheters are characterized by the ease of insertion and low complication rates, especially when placed under radiologic guidance. The image-guided placement is particularly useful in patients with certain risk factors, minimizing the rate of potential adverse events.

REFERENCES

1. Kalso E. A short history of central venous catheterization. *Acta Anaesth Scand* 1985;81(suppl):7–10.
2. Keeri-Szanto M. The subclavian vein, a constant and convenient intravenous injection site. *Arch Surg* 1956; 72:179–181.
3. Hermosura B, Vanags L, Dickey MW. Measurement of pressure during intravenous therapy. *JAMA* 1966;195: 181.
4. Kenney PR, Dorfman GS, Denny DF. Percutaneous inferior vena cava cannulation for long term parenteral access. *Surgery* 1985;97:602–605.
5. Crummy AB, Carlson P, McDermott JC, et al. Percutaneous transhepatic placement of a Hickman catheter. *AJR* 1989;153:1317–1318.
6. Kaufman JK, Greenfield AJ, Fitzpatrick GF. Transhepatic cannulation of the inferior vena cava. *JVIR* 1991; 2:331–334.
7. Schwab S, Besarab A, Beathard G, et al. *NKF-DOQI clinical practice guidelines for vascular access.* New York: National Kidney Foundation, 1997.
8. Openshaw KL, Picus D, Hicks ME, et al. Interventional radiologic placement of Hohn central venous catheters: results and complications in 100 consecutive patients. *JVIR* 1994;5:111–115.
9. Raad I, Davis S, Becker M, et al. Low infection rate and long durability of nontunneled silastic catheters. *Arch Intern Med* 1993;153:1791–1796.
10. Namyslowski J. Temporary acute care central venous access devices. *Semin Intervent Radiol* 1998;15:253–258.
11. Andris DA, Krzywda EA. Central venous access. Clinical practice issues. *Nurs Clin North Am* 1997;32: 719–740.
12. Whitman ED. Complications associated with the use of central venous access devices. *Curr Probl Surg* 1996; 33:312–369.
13. Mansfield PF, Hohn DC, Fornage BD, et al. Complications and failures of subclavian-vein catheterization. *N Engl J Med* 1994;331:1735–1738.
14. Ray CE, Shenoy SS. Radiologic placement of central venous access devices in patients with thrombocytopenia. *Radiology* 1997;204:97–99.
15. Denny DF. The role of the radiologist in long-term central-vein access. *Radiology* 1992;185:637–638.
16. Teichgraber UKM, Benter T, Gebel M, Manns MP. A sonographically guided technique for central venous access. *AJR* 1997;169:731–733.
17. Denys BG, Uretsky BF. Anatomical variations of internal jugular vein location: Impact on central venous access. *Crit Care Med* 1991;19:1516–1519.
18. Farrell J, Gellens M. Ultrasound-guided cannulation versus the landmark-guided technique for acute haemodialysis access. *Nephrol Dial Transplant* 1997; 12:1234–1237.
19. Ledgerwood AM, Saxe JM, Lucas CE. Venous access devices: a review. *Surg Ann* 1993;25:45–57.
20. Denys BG, Uretsky BF, Reddy PS. Ultrasound-assisted cannulation of the internal jugular vein. A prospective comparison with the external landmark-guided technique. *Circulation* 1993;87:1557–1562.
21. Agee KR, Balk RA. Central venous catheterization in the critically ill patient. *Crit Care Clin* 1992;8: 677–686.
22. Sznajder JI, Zveibil FR, Bitterman H, et al. Central vein catheterization. Failure and complications by three percutaneous approaches. *Arch Intern Med* 1986; 146:259–261.
23. Lewis CA, Allen TE, Burke DR, et al. Quality improvement guidelines for central venous access. *JVIR* 1997;8:475–479.
24. Trottier SJ, Veremakis C, O'Brien J, et al. Femoral deep vein thrombosis associated with central venous catheterization: results from a prospective, randomized trial. *Crit Care Med* 1995;23:52–59.
25. Collignon P, Soni N, Pearson I, et al. Sepsis associated with central vein catheters in critically ill patients. *Int Care Med* 1988;14:227–231.
26. Gil RT, Kruse JA, Thill-Baharozian MC, et al. Triple- vs single-lumen central venous catheters. A prospective study in critically ill population. *Arch Intern Med* 1989;149:1139–1143.
27. Pearson ML. Guideline for prevention of intravascular device-related infections. *Infect Control Hosp Epidemiol* 1996;17:438–473.
28. Trerotola SO, Johnson MS, Harris VJ, et al. Outcome of tunneled hemodialysis catheters placed via the right internal jugular vein by interventional radiologists. *Radiology* 1997;203:489–495.

Central Venous Access
Edited by Charles E. Ray, Jr.
Lippincott Williams & Wilkins, Philadelphia © 2001.

6

Implantable Port Devices

Chieh-Min Fan, MD

Department of Radiology, Massachusetts General Hospital; Harvard Medical School,
Boston, Massachusetts 02114

Commonly referred to as chest ports and porta-caths, central venous ports are long-term venous access devices that are distinguished by the fact that they are implanted completely subcutaneously. Among various types of long-term venous access devices, ports arguably provide access for low flow rate exchanges with the least amount of inconvenience and restriction to patient life-style and activity. When unaccessed, the entire device is sequestered from the extracorporeal environment, providing better cosmesis while permitting the patient to shower, swim, and pursue physical activities without the fear of accidental dislodgement of the device.

Chest ports are particularly appropriate for patients in whom infrequent intermittent access is required (e.g., monthly chemotherapy). Because accessing a port requires percutaneous needle insertion through the patient's skin, leaving a port chronically accessed can lead to patient discomfort and increase the risk of pocket infection. For these reasons, ports are not the device of choice for prolonged continuous infusions such as parenteral nutrition or chronic dobutamine therapy. In such situations, a peripherally inserted central catheter line or tunneled catheter would be a preferable device (1).

Traditionally placed by surgeons, over the past decade placement of chest ports has become standard practice in many interventional radiology practices. Advantages of radiologic versus surgical placement include controlled venipuncture under venographic or sonographic guidance, ease of scheduling, lower cost, and definitive final catheter positioning. In addition, fluoroscopic techniques permit port placement in patients with difficult anatomy due to central venous occlusion, and facilitate use of alternative access routes such as translumbar and transhepatic placement. Initial concern of potentially higher device infection rates with placement outside the operating room has not been validated in practice (2).

DEVICE DESIGN

Chest ports are available in either single- or double-lumen designs, and in a spectrum of sizes to accommodated differences in patient size and body habitus (3). Despite minor variations of design, all chest ports have the same three main mechanical components: a port reservoir, catheter, and connector that prevents detachment of the catheter from the port (Fig. 6.1A). The port reservoir is constructed from either plastic or metal (stainless steel or titanium), and has a centrally positioned silicon diaphragm (4). Accessing the device involves puncturing the diaphragm with a noncoring needle (e.g., Huber needle), and confirmation of successful access of the reservoir by aspiration of blood. The silicon diaphragm is typically designed to withstand 2,000 to 4,000 punctures during the lifetime of the device (5) (Fig. 6.1B).

Chest port catheters range in size from 3 to 12 French (Fr), and are constructed from silicon

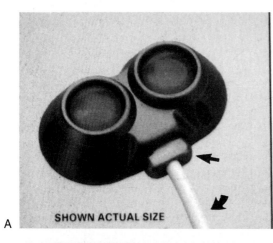

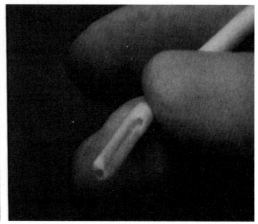

A

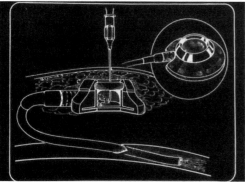

B

FIG. 6.1. A: Full-size dual-lumen chest port demonstrating the three structural components: reservoir with silicon diaphragms (*arrowhead*), connector (*arrow*), and catheter (*curved arrow*). **B:** Schematic diagram of Huber needle accessing an implanted port.

or polyurethane. The catheter is usually fitted onto the port reservoir and locked into this position with a connector. The connector design varies among different manufacturers and includes screw-on lock mechanisms as well as snap-on connectors. Ports with preattached catheters are also available.

dual-lumen ports require a larger pocket for implantation and have larger catheters with an associated higher risk of venous thrombosis. When not in use, two lumens instead of one must be periodically flushed. For these reasons, more lumens are not always preferable, and an

DEVICE SELECTION

Although varying slightly in design features (Fig. 6.2), the commercially available chest ports are comparable in function and clinical outcome. However, certain parameters require consideration when selecting a device for a specific patient.

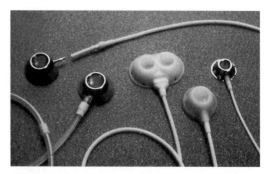

FIG. 6.2. Examples of different models of chest ports.

Number of Lumens

Ports are available in single- and double-lumen designs. Although functionally similar, attempt should be made to match the patient's infusion needs to the number of lumens of the device. Multidrug regimens involving incompatible agents warrant dual-lumen devices, whereas single-drug regimens or access for intermittent blood sampling are adequately served by a single-lumen device.

Device Size

Both single- and double-lumen port reservoirs are available in full-size and smaller low-profile designs. Appropriate sizing of the device to a patient's body habitus is essential to facilitate accessing the device and to prevent skin complications. Oversizing the device results in tension in the overlying skin, which can lead to skin erosion over the port; undersizing the device makes the device difficult to locate by palpation and hence difficult to access. Most patients of average body habitus are adequately served with low-profile ports. Patients with a large amount of adipose tissue or redundant chest wall tissue are better served with full-size devices. Due to the thinner skin and subcutaneous tissues in the arm, low-profile or mini ports are preferred for use as arm ports.

ACCESS ROUTES

Conventional access routes for chest port placement include the internal jugular and subclavian veins. The jugular approach has been shown to be associated with a significantly lower incidence of central venous obstruction (6–8), and is therefore the preferred access route for most operators. In patients with central venous occlusions, alternative routes such as translumbar or transhepatic placement can be used (9–11).

Many factors should be considered when choosing an access site. In general, ports should be placed on the side opposite to the disease process to avoid obstructing or creating a surgical incision inside a radiation field. Dermatologic problems such as skin infections, postradiation changes, or burns mandate contralateral placement, as do central venous occlusions. In the absence of other extenuating circumstances, the port is placed on the side contralateral to the patient's dominant hand so that potential complications will result in less functional impairment.

PORT INSERTION TECHNIQUE

Patient Preparation

Routine preplacement screening blood work includes prothrombin time (PT), partial prothrombin time, platelet count, blood urea nitrogen, and creatinine. Port insertion is a minor surgical procedure involving an incision and tissue disruption, so it is important that coagulation parameters are normal (PT <14, platelets >50,000/dL) to avoid bleeding complications

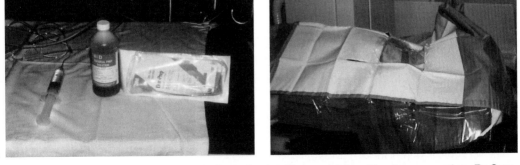

A   B

FIG. 6.3. A: Alcohol preparation and iodinated paint (Duraprep) for skin site preparation. **B:** Complete draping of the patient to ensure sterility of the operative field.

and pocket hematomas, which increase the risk for infection. Patients are asked to wear a cap and mask during the procedure. Placement is performed under conscious sedation with midozalam and fentanyl, which requires that the patient not eat for 4 to 6 hours prior to the procedure.

Operator Preparation

The operator should wear a cap and mask and follow meticulous sterile technique, including a 5-minute full surgical scrub prior to performing the procedure.

Skin Site Preparation

Skin at the insertion site is widely prepared from the mandible to the nipple craniocaudally, and from the sternum to the mid-axillary line laterally. At our institution, a double preparation with betadine and alcohol scrub is performed, followed by application of an iodine paint with long-acting bacteriostatic properties (Duraprep, 3M Health Care, St. Paul, MN, U.S.A.) (Fig. 6.3A). The patient is then covered completely with sterile drapes, leaving only the insertion site exposed (Fig. 6.3B).

Establishing Access

Jugular Approach

The jugular vein is punctured under sonographic guidance using a 21-gauge needle and 0.018-inch mandrill wire (micropuncture kit, Cook, Inc., Bloomington, IN, U.S.A.). A 5 Fr introducer is inserted and the wire is exchanged for a 0.035-inch working wire that is positioned into the inferior vena cava. The venipuncture site is sequentially dilated to admit an appropriate sized peel-away sheath, through which the port catheter is advanced.

Subclavian Approach

The subclavian vein is localized venographically and under fluoroscopic observation, and the vein is accessed using the micropuncture

system described above. Care is taken to keep the anterior first rib beneath the needle tip at all times, thus essentially eliminating the risk of pneumothorax (Fig. 6.4A). The needle is advanced until it meets the first rib, and then is withdrawn while continually aspirating until blood return is achieved. The mandrill wire is then advanced, the introducer is placed, and the wire is exchanged for a 0.035-inch working wire over which the peel-away sheath is placed. The catheter is then inserted and the peel-away sheath removed (Fig. 6.4B-D). A hemostat is placed over the catheter to prevent reflux of blood and catheter clotting while the port pocket is created.

Arm Approach

Basilic or cephalic veins are accessed under venographic or sonographic guidance, and sheath insertion proceeds as outlined above.

Pocket Creation

The port is placed on the skin to assess incision size and location (Fig. 6.4E). The skin and subcutaneous tissues at the pocket site are infiltrated with 2% xylocaine local anesthesia (Fig. 6.4F). Using a scalpel with a no. 15 blade, an incision is made through the dermis to expose the subcutaneous fat (Fig. 6.4G). Using blunt dissection, the tissues are gently separated to create a small pocket under the skin (Fig. 6.4H and I). Care should be taken to keep at least 1 cm thickness of tissue between the port and the skin to prevent skin erosion over the port. The pocket should be checked periodically for any active bleeding. Bleeding vessels should be isolated and controlled either by cauterization or ligation. Once the pocket is created, the port should be fitted inside to check for positioning and size. It should insert easily without the need for excessive manipulation, and should not protrude into the incision.

Port Assembly and Implantation

Once the pocket is created, the catheter is tunneled to the pocket using a blunt instrument

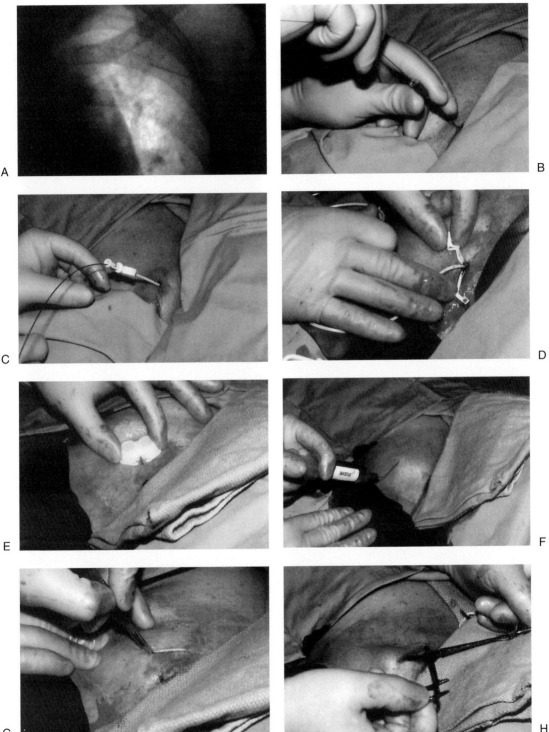

FIG. 6.4. Sequential steps for chest port placement. **A:** Subclavian vein puncture using first rib technique, taking care to keep the anterior first rib between the needle tip and lung at all times. **B:** Passing the 0.018-inch mandril wire. **C:** Exchange for a working 0.035-inch wire and peel-away sheath. **D:** Insertion of catheter and removal of peel-away sheath. **E:** Assessing position and length of incision. **F:** Anesthetizing the soft tissues prior to pocket creation. **G:** Incising the skin. **H:** Spreading the soft tissues with a blunt instrument.

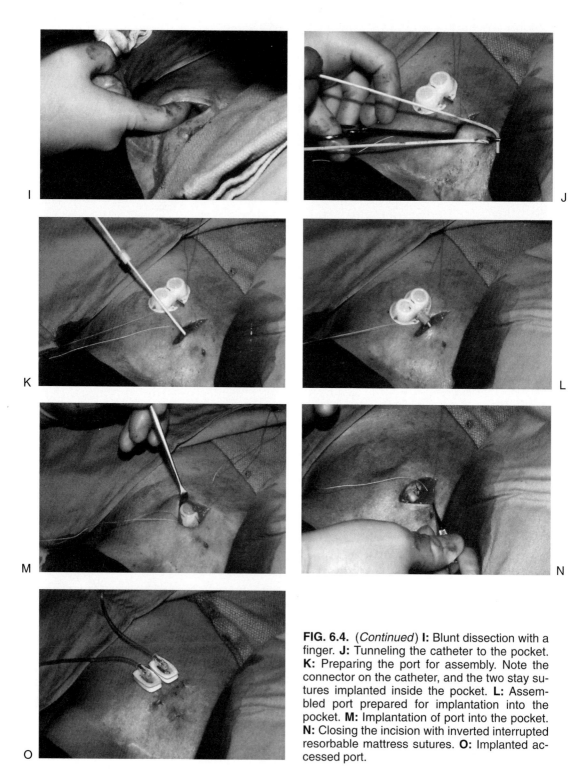

FIG. 6.4. (*Continued*) **I:** Blunt dissection with a finger. **J:** Tunneling the catheter to the pocket. **K:** Preparing the port for assembly. Note the connector on the catheter, and the two stay sutures implanted inside the pocket. **L:** Assembled port prepared for implantation into the pocket. **M:** Implantation of port into the pocket. **N:** Closing the incision with inverted interrupted resorbable mattress sutures. **O:** Implanted accessed port.

(Fig. 6.4J). Two resorbable 3–0 vicryl stay sutures are placed into the medial and lateral aspects of the pocket base, and run through the two anchoring holes adjacent to the stem of the port. These stay sutures prevent rotation of the port within the pocket; if the port fits snugly in the pocket, the stay sutures are optional (Figs. 6.4J and K). The connector is placed over the external end of the catheter, and the catheter is pulled back to position the tip in the high right atrium. Of note, patients with mobile chest tissue may demonstrate 3 to 6 cm of cephalad retraction of the catheter when assuming the upright position (Fig. 6.5). By examining the patient prior to the procedure, this positional change can be predicted and remedied by initially positioning the catheter deeper into the right atrium. Once the tip position is determined, the excess external catheter is trimmed. The catheter is connected to the port reservoir, and the components are secured together with the connector (Fig. 6.4L). Using a Huber needle, the port is accessed and patency confirmed with aspiration of blood. The device is flushed with 5 to 10 mL of 100 U/mL heparin solution while observing carefully for any leakage at the connection. Once integrity of the port connection is confirmed, the entire device is gently manipulated into the pocket, and the stay sutures are tied securely to anchor the device to the base of the pocket (Fig. 6.4M).

Incision Closure

The incision is closed in layers with resorbable 3–0 vicryl interrupted inverted mattress sutures subcutaneously, and either steri-strips or interrupted 5–0 ethilon sutures for the skin. If the port is to be used immediately, a Huber access system is inserted immediately after skin closure. A sterile occlusive dressing is applied (Fig. 6.4N and O).

Postprocedural Management

The original dressing is left undisturbed and the patient is asked to refrain from showering for the initial 48 hours. After the first 2 days, the patient may shower and change the dressing daily until the incision is fully healed. Any nonresorbable skin closure sutures may be removed after 10 days. Once the site is fully healed (14 days), the patient may shower and swim. All port lumens should be flushed with 5 to 10 mL of 100 U/mL heparin solution after each use, and monthly when not in use. A more detailed description is provided in Chapter 10.

Arm Ports

The placement of an arm port is analogous to chest port placement. Because the arm is a more mobile structure, however, traction forces on the catheter may be more pronounced. To minimize these forces, the pocket is created in a cephalad instead of caudad direction, forcing the catheter to make a U-turn configuration (Fig. 6.6).

Port Removal

Reasons for port removal include completion of therapy, device malfunction, and device infection. Removal is generally a simple procedure that does not require conscious sedation. The port pocket is anesthetized with 2% xylocaine, and an incision is made across the cephalad aspect of the pocket or over the prior port insertion incision. Using blunt dissection, the fibrous capsule of the pocket is entered, the port is freed from the underlying tissues, and the device is removed as a single unit. Uninfected pockets are closed in two layers, as is done during port placement. Infected pockets cannot be closed primarily; instead, the pocket is packed with sterile gauze and the wound is covered with a loose nonocclusive dressing. The packing is changed daily until the wound heals by secondary intent.

OUTCOMES

Although more costly and more complicated to insert, implantable ports provide long-term venous access with lower early and late complication rates than tunneled catheters. Early and late complications for implantable ports are

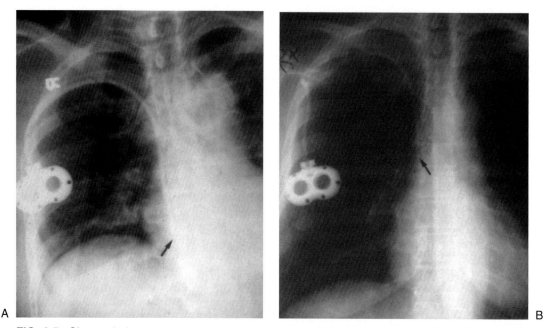

A   B

FIG. 6.5. Change in intravascular position of the catheter tip (*arrow*) in supine **(A)** versus upright **(B)** position due to retraction from soft tissue movement.

2.3% and 10.6 %, respectively, compared with 10.7% and 37.6 % for tunneled lines (12). Several large series examining the outcome of surgically placed ports demonstrated a 6% to 11% rate of infection (sepsis and pocket infections combined), a 5% rate for catheter compromise at the level of the clavicle (pinch off syndrome), 8% to 10% rates of catheter-related venous thrombosis, and 1% to 2% rates of procedure-related pneumothorax (13–17). Overall, late complications result in port revision or explantation prior to completion of treatment in 11% to 13% of surgically placed ports (13–17).

Outcomes of radiologically placed ports compare favorably with the surgical experience. With the advantage of fluoroscopic guidance and advanced angiographic techniques, the overall technical success of radiologic placement approaches 100%. The incidence of infectious complications is 5% to 6%, procedure-related pneumothorax 1% to 2%, catheter-related thrombosis 5% to 10%, and overall early device removal 8% to 13% (18–20).

COMPLICATIONS

Complications related to implantable ports can be categorized into early complications associated with the placement procedure (pneumothorax, central venous perforation, pocket hematomas, early infection) and late complications (pericatheter thrombosis, fibrin sheath formation, late pocket infection, catheter fragmentation, catheter migration, and port thrombosis). Complications specific to ports or seen more commonly with ports are discussed in detail in Chapter 14.

Infection

The incidence of port infection following radiologic placement is approximately 5%, comparable with the rates seen with surgical placement. The most commonly implicated pathogens are *Staphylococcus epidermidis* and *S. aureus,* which account for 50% to 75%, and *Candida* fungal infections, which account for

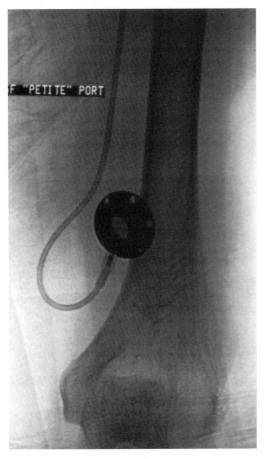

FIG. 6.6. Arm port orientation.

involves removal of the device and packing of the wound as described above.

Catheter Migration

Migration of the catheter into other central venous structures can result from flow dynamics and cardiac motion within the central veins, or from retraction forces from soft tissue movement outside the chest (23). Patients with abundant or highly mobile chest wall soft tissues have a higher risk of catheter retraction; this is especially true for tunneled or implantable devices (Fig. 6.7). Catheters that are too short (above the atrial caval junction) have a higher likelihood of migration into the contralateral jugular or brachiocephalic veins. If the catheter is still intravascular, repositioning can be performed via snaring from a femoral approach. If mobile chest wall tissue is the inciting problem, an arm port may provide more stable device positioning. Care should be taken prior to placement of the device to be certain that the port is not placed in excessive and mobile soft tissues of the chest. Placement of the port in a more

about 10%. Port infections can be subdivided into catheter colonization and true pocket infections. The former typically present with rigors and bacteremia during infusion through the port. Definitive diagnosis is made using quantitative cultures: a colony count of the sample drawn from the port that is greater than ten times the colony count from a peripherally drawn blood sample indicates a catheter-related infection (21,22). True pocket infections present as erythema, tenderness, and swelling around the device, occasionally with fluctuance around the pocket. Whereas catheter infections can sometimes be salvaged with antibiotic therapy, pocket infections cannot be irradicated with antibiotics alone, and definitive treatment

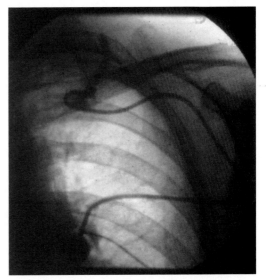

FIG. 6.7. Migration of the catheter completely extravascularly due to excessive movement of chest wall soft tissues.

medial location can help prevent this, as can measures such as taping the breast tissue down prior to preparing the patient.

Twiddler's Syndrome

Twiddler's syndrome consists of inversion of the port in the pocket following placement; it is so named because of the proclivity for some patients to play with their ports postimplantation. Typically, inversion can only occur in the early postprocedure period prior to formation of the fibrous capsule around the port reservoir. Prevention of the syndrome can easily be accomplished either by sizing the port pocket appropriately or by placing stay sutures around the post base. Occasionally, the port can be reinverted by external manipulations, but definitive therapy frequently requires opening the incision and correcting the port position.

SUMMARY

Interventional radiologists have assumed an increasingly dominant role in the placement of venous access devices, including implantable ports. Radiologic placement has the advantage of controlled venipuncture, ease of scheduling, lower cost, and precise final positioning of the device. Complications of radiologic versus surgical placement are comparable.

REFERENCES

1. Reed WP, Newman KA, Wade JC. Choosing an appropriate implantable device for long-term venous access. *Eur J Cancer Clin Oncol* 1989;25:1383–1391.
2. McGann GM. Long-term venous access service based in the barium room. *Br J Radiol* 1995;68:590–592.
3. Hadaway LC. Comparison of vascular access devices. *Semin Oncol Nurs* 1995;11:154–166.
4. Shellock FG, Morisoli S, Canal E. MR procedures and biomedical implants: materials and devices. 1993 update. *Radiology* 1993;189:587–599.
5. Ahmad I, Ray CE. Radiological placement of venous access ports. *Semin Int Radiol* 1998;15:259–272.
6. Spinowitz BS, Galler M, Golden RA, et al. Subclavian vein stenosis as a complication of subclavian vein catheterization for hemodialysis. *Arch Intern Med* 1987;147:305–307.
7. Vanherweghem JL, Yassine T, Goldman M, et al. Subclavian vein thrombosis: a frequent complication of subclavian vein cannulation for hemodialysis. *Clin Nephrol* 1986;26:235–238.
8. Cimochowski GE, Worley E, Rutherford WE, et al. Superiority of internal jugular over subclavian access for temporary dialysis. *Nephron* 1990;54:154–161.
9. Lund GB, Trerotola SO, Scheel PJ. Percutaneous translumbar inferior vena cava cannulation for hemodialysis. *Am J Kidney Dis* 1995;25:732–737.
10. Denny DF, Dorfman GS, Greenwood LH, et al. Translumbar inferior vena cava Hickman catheter placement for total parenteral nutrition. *AJR* 1987;148:621–622.
11. Kaufman JA, Greenfield AJ, Fitzpatrick GF. Transhepatic cannulation of the inferior vena cava. *JVIR* 1991;2:331–334.
12. Pullyblank AM, Tanner AG, Carey PD, et al. Comparison between peripherally implanted ports and externally sited catheters for long-term venous access. *Ann R Coll Surg Engl* 1994;76:33–38.
13. Lemmers NWM, Gels ME, Sluijfer DT, et al. Complications of venous access ports in 132 patients with disseminated testicular cancer treated with polychemotherapy. *J Clin Oncol* 1996;14:2916–2922.
14. Rubie H, Juricic M, Claeyssens S, et al. Morbidity using subcutaneous ports and efficacy of vancomycin flushing in cancer. *Arch Dis Child* 1995;72:325–329.
15. Koonings PP, Given FT. Long term experience with a totally implanted catheter system in gynecological oncologic patients. *J Am Coll Surg* 1994;178:164–178.
16. Harvey WH, Pick TE, Reed K, et al. A prospective evaluation of the port-a-cath implantable venous access system in chronically ill adults and children. *Surg Gynecol Obstet* 1989;169:495–500.
17. Puig-LaCalle J, Sanchez SL, Serra EP, et al. Totally implanted device for long-term intravenous chemotherapy: experience in 123 adult patients with solid neoplasms. *J Surg Oncol* 1996;62:273–278.
18. Denny DF. Placement and management of long-term central venous access catheters and ports. *AJR* 1993;161: 385–393.
19. Morris SL, Jaques PF, Mauro MA. Radiology-assisted placement of implantable subcutaneous infusion ports for long-term venous access. *Radiology* 1992;184:149–151.
20. Simpson KR, Hovesepian DM, Picus D. Interventional radiologic placement of chest wall ports: results and complications in 161 consecutive placements. *JVIR* 1997;8:189–195.
21. Benezra D, Kiehn TE, Golod JW, et al. Prospective study of infections in indwelling central venous catheters using quantitative blood cultures. *Am J Med* 1988;85:495–498.
22. Weightman NC, Simpson M, Speller CE, et al. Bacteremia related to indwelling central venous catheters: prevention, diagnosis, and treatment. *Eur J Clin Microbiol Infect Dis* 1988;7:125–129.
23. Rasuli P, Hammond DI, Peterkin IR. Spontaneous intrajugular migration of long-term central venous access catheters. *Radiology* 1992;182:822–824.

Central Venous Access
Edited by Charles E. Ray, Jr.
Lippincott Williams & Wilkins, Philadelphia © 2001.

7

Tunneled Catheters

Guido M. Scatorchia, MD

Department of Radiology, Denver Health Medical Center;
University of Colorado Health Sciences Center, Denver, Colorado 80204

Venous access for patients requiring long-term intravenous therapy has undergone great advances over the past three decades. Prior to 1970, indwelling peripheral catheters were attempted but were found to be cumbersome and difficult to maintain for extended periods of time. Surgically placed arteriovenous fistulae were one solution to the problem of prolonged venous access, but fistulae require a 6-week maturation period before they can be used. In addition, fistulae were found to have a high failure rate when used for vascular access in patients other than those with chronic renal failure. Another form of arteriovenous shunt developed by Thomas, which involved the use of an external silastic catheter, likewise met with little success (1). Tunneled central venous catheters came to be used commonly in the early 1970s. In 1973, Broviac et al. published the first paper describing the use of an implantable silicone catheter in patients requiring long-term total parenteral nutrition (TPN) (2). Use of this catheter made it possible for patients to receive intravenous therapy as outpatients. The silastic-silicone catheter was found to have a relatively low rate of infection with long intravascular dwell times, and good patency when intermittently flushed with dilute heparin solution.

In his original article, Broviac recommended the use of the implantable catheter solely for parenteral nutrition. Once it was demonstrated that tunneled catheters could be used safely, other indications became apparent. The clinical utility of the catheter was expanded in 1975 when Hickman modified the Broviac catheter by enlarging its internal diameter from 1.0 mm to 1.6 mm (3). In 1980, Ponsky and Gauderer published an article that supported expanded applications of the tunneled silastic catheter, including intravenous access for patients requiring prolonged courses of antibiotic therapy and those with malignant processes requiring frequent intravenous therapy (3). Since then, the indications for long-term venous access have broadened even more and include patients with hematologic disorders requiring frequent blood product infusions and (once larger bore catheters were developed) hemodialysis patients and blood stem cell transplant patients.

A wide range of tunneled catheter sizes is currently available. The smallest Broviac catheter measures 2.7 French (Fr) (Bard Access Systems, Salt Lake City, UT, U.S.A.) and is used in the pediatric population; the largest catheters measure 13.5 Fr (e.g., Optiflow, Bard) and are used when higher flow rates are required, as in hemodialysis and apheresis patients. Larger catheters are available with one to three lumens, the choice of lumen number depending on the intended use of the catheter. Regardless of the size of the catheter or the number of lumens, all tunneled catheters share several characteristics. Most tunneled catheters are made either from a material known as silastic, which is a silicone rubber based material, or from polyurethane. These materials have been consistently used because they are soft, durable, and biologically inert and have a lower incidence of thrombotic complications when compared with less pliable materials such as polyvinylchloride (4). All tunneled catheters are placed in the same fashion, with creation of a subcutaneous tunnel that connects the venipuncture site with the site where the catheter exits the skin. All catheters also have a Dacron cuff that is positioned within the subcutaneous tunnel to allow for connective tissue ingrowth; this connective tissue functions both in anchoring the catheter and providing a theoretical mechanical barrier to infection. Some catheters have used an additional silver-impregnated collagen cuff (Vitacuff; Vitaphore, San Carlos, CA) to help decrease infection rates, but the benefit of the second cuff has not been definitively demonstrated (5–9). At least one investigator has demonstrated that the silver-impregnated cuff may impede the fibrotic reaction elicited by the Dacron cuff (10). For this reason, many catheter manufacturers currently separate the cuffs on the catheter shaft.

Originally, tunneled catheters were surgically placed in the operating room using either a blind venipuncture or cutdown technique. Over the past decade there has been a gradual transition from surgical placement of these devices to placement by interventional radiologists in the radiology department. The transition is well supported by many studies comparing the outcome, cost, and efficacy of radiologic versus surgical placement of tunneled catheters (11–14). A recent large series examined the success and immediate complication rates in 880 consecutive radiologically-placed tunneled central venous catheters. In this study, venous access was successful in 99.4% of patients, the immediate complication rate was 4.0%, and no major complications were reported (15).

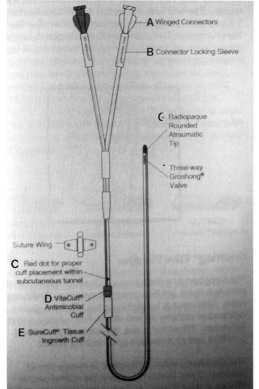

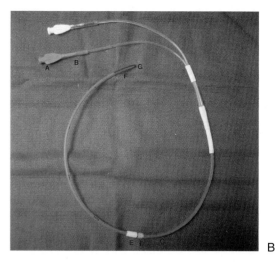

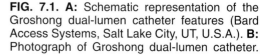

FIG. 7.1. A: Schematic representation of the Groshong dual-lumen catheter features (Bard Access Systems, Salt Lake City, UT, U.S.A.). **B:** Photograph of Groshong dual-lumen catheter.

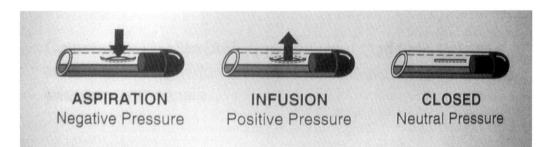

ASPIRATION
Negative Pressure

INFUSION
Positive Pressure

CLOSED
Neutral Pressure

FIG. 7.2. Schematic representation of the three-position Groshong valve. The valve allows fluid infusion and blood aspiration. When not in use, the valve restricts blood backflow and air embolism by remaining closed. The Groshong valve is designed to remain closed between pressures of -7 and +80 mm Hg; therefore, at normal central venous pressures, the valve remains closed. If the catheter is aspirated, pulling the valve inward, it must be flushed forward to allow the valve to return to its normal closed position.

CATHETER TYPES

Tunneled catheters can be broadly divided into two groups: the Hickman and Broviac type catheters, and the larger dual lumen catheters used for hemodialysis and apheresis. The larger bore 13.5 Fr catheters are used when greater flow rates are required and are discussed more fully in Chapter 8. Broviac and Hickman catheters range in size from 2.7 to 12.5 Fr.

Aside from size, Broviac and Hickman catheters are similar in design. Broviac catheters are single-lumen catheters that range in size from 2.7 to 6.6 Fr and are designed for use in the pediatric population. The external and tunneled segments of the catheter are larger to help prevent breakage, whereas the intravenous segment is tapered in caliber. The Hickman catheter ranges in size from 7.0 to 12.5 Fr and is available in single-, double-, and triple-lumen configurations.

Currently, the most common tunneled catheters used in adults are the Hickman and Groshong catheters. The Groshong catheter is available as small as 7.0 Fr and, like the Hickman catheter, is available with one to three lumens (Fig. 7.1). The distinction between the Groshong and Hickman catheters is that the Groshong has a longitudinal slit valve at its distal tip (Fig. 7.2). The tip opens outward during positive pressure infusions and inward for negative pressure aspirations, and remains closed when not in use. This design has some theoreti-

cal advantages, including a reduction in the need for routine daily flushing, thereby reducing daily care costs, and a decrease in the risk of mechanical and infectious complications; in actuality, these have not been substantiated. In a study among pediatric oncology patients that compared Hickman and Groshong catheters, Groshong catheters required more frequent removal for mechanical complications, more frequent daily flushings for preventing the reflux of blood into the lumen, and a greater number of urokinase instillations for lumenal clotting. As a result, the daily maintenance cost was found to be comparable with that of the Hickman catheter (16). In studies of nursing and patient satisfaction, the greatest global satisfaction was found with the Hickman catheter; there were more flow-related problems and a higher incidence of catheter thrombosis with the Groshong catheter (17,18). No study reported to date has demonstrated Groshong catheters to have a lower rate of catheter-related infection, and infection rates have been shown to be comparable between Hickman and Groshong catheters (19).

PREPROCEDURAL CONSIDERATIONS

As discussed above, the indications for tunneled central venous access include, but are not limited to, those patients requiring chemotherapy, TPN, prolonged antibiotic therapy (as required in osteomyelitis and subacute bacterial endocarditis), long-term blood product replacement (patients with hematologic disorders such as myelodysplastic disorders, refractory anemias, hemoglobinopathies, and clotting disorders), hemodialysis, or apheresis. The recent increasing popularity of nontunneled silastic catheters has only slightly challenged the concept of the tunneled catheter. Both the peripherally inserted central catheter (PICC) and the Hohn catheter (placed centrally via the internal jugular or subclavian veins) have been demonstrated to be safe for intermediate-term use. These catheters are finding their niche in situations where access has a well-defined end point of up to 6 to 8 weeks. To date, no study has examined the long-term use of nontunneled silastic catheters as compared to tunneled catheters; at our institution, patients requiring therapy for longer than 8 weeks receive either a tunneled catheter or an implantable port. PICCs and Hohn catheters are discussed in more detail in Chapters 5 and 9.

The strongest contraindication to tunneled catheter placement is active infection. At our institution, if a patient is febrile or has an elevated white blood cell count, a tunneled catheter is not placed until he or she has been afebrile for 24 to 48 hours or until the white blood cell count normalizes. If the patient is bacteremic with positive blood cultures, serial cultures are obtained until a negative culture is drawn. If central access is required until a time appropriate for tunneled catheter placement, a temporary catheter is placed.

Disorders of clotting are a relative contraindication to placing a tunneled catheter. We obtain a platelet count and a coagulation profile on all patients scheduled for tunneled catheter placement. A platelet count greater than 50,000/mm^3 is preferred; for counts less than this, platelets are transfused accordingly. One unit of random donor platelet concentrate generally elevates the platelet count by 5,000 to 10,000/mm^3 in the absence of active platelet consumption. A unit dose of 10 units of platelets contains approximately 500 mL of plasma, which roughly equals 2 units of fresh frozen plasma (FFP). Previously allosensitized pa-

tients may require single-donor human leukocyte antigen (HLA)-matched platelets to prevent accelerated immune destruction. An international normalized ratio (INR) of 1.3 or less is preferable for catheter placement. Abnormalities are corrected with FFP, which represents a good source of the intrinsic clotting factors. Each unit of FFP elevates the level of clotting factors by 2% to 3%. For patients who are taking coumadin, coumadin is discontinued and a heparin drip is instituted to maintain anticoagulation while the INR is allowed to normalize; 2 hours prior to the procedure, the heparin is stopped and catheter placement is performed through the heparin window.

Patients are instructed to take nothing by mouth for 6 hours prior to the procedure in anticipation of the need for intravenous sedation during catheter placement. Monitored administration of a combination of an anxiolytic and an analgesic is usually sufficient to make the procedure relatively comfortable for the patient. In our department, a combination of the short-acting benzodiazepine midazolam (Versed, Roche Laboratories) and the narcotic fentanyl are routinely used. For healthy adults under 60 years of age, an initial dose of 1 mg of midazolam is given intravenously. Three to five minutes should be allowed to fully evaluate the sedative effect; additional medication can then be titrated to achieve the desired level of sedation. A total dose of greater than 5 mg is not usually necessary to reach the desired end point. In older or debilitated patients, lower doses should be used. Fentanyl is also a short-acting agent. It is 50 times more potent than morphine, but it has a less sedative effect than other narcotics. In young healthy adults, an initial dose of 50 µg is given and, as with midazolam, can be titrated to the desired effect based on the patient's needs during the procedure. Fentanyl is contraindicated in patients on monoamine oxidase inhibitors. For respiratory depression and overdoses of fentanyl, naloxone can be administered at a dose of 0.4 mg intravenously. Versed and fentanyl are usually given concurrently because they have a synergistic effect.

The issue of prophylactic antibiotic administration remains controversial. There remains little data to support the routine administration of prophylactic antibiotics for tunneled catheter placement. A randomized, controlled study by Ranson et al. demonstrated no effect on the rate of catheter-related sepsis in cancer patients when given vancomycin at the time of catheter placement (20). Another randomized, controlled study by McKee et al. also found no effect of prophylactic vancomycin on the rate of catheter infection in a population of patients receiving parenteral nutrition (21). Many operators continue to support the use of prophylactic antibiotics, arguing that infection necessitates catheter removal and that a course of intravenous antibiotics may justify prophylaxis (22). Review of the literature provides no consensus as to the resolution of this issue; further studies are required to clarify how to best protect patients without overusing antibiotics, causing selective overgrowth of drug-resistant strains of bacteria.

For tunneled catheter placement, the interventional radiology suite is treated as an operating room with regard to sterile technique. The patient and all staff in the room should wear surgical caps and masks. The operator and assistant perform a full surgical scrub prior to gowning and gloving. The skin site is widely prepared with a full surgical scrub. At our institution, a Betadyne surgical preparation (Purdue Frederick Co., Norwalk, CT, U.S.A.) is used; an alternative preparation is chlorhexadine (e.g., Hibiclens, Zeneca Pharmaceuticals, Wilmington, DE, U.S.A.). Multiple studies have demonstrated that long-term central venous access catheters placed by interventional radiologists have infection rates comparable to catheters placed by surgeons in the operating room (23–27). To maintain this low rate of periprocedural catheter infection, strict adherence to sterile technique must be maintained.

CATHETER INSERTION

Several factors come into play when selecting the venous access site. Patient history is an important consideration. If there is a history of multiple prior central venous catheters, venous patency should be evaluated prior to catheter placement by venography, duplex Doppler ul-

trasonography, or magnetic resonance venography. Extremity swelling also may provide a clue to central venous thrombosis, and should be evaluated in a similar manner. Other factors such as a history of surgery, radiation therapy, infection, scarring, or dermatologic disorder also influence selection of an access site. Patients often express a preference to have the catheter placed on their nondominant side, yet another practical consideration in selecting an access site.

Allowing for these considerations, the most common venous access routes in adults are the internal jugular vein (IJV) and subclavian vein (SCV), with the IJV having several advantages over the SCV. It is well documented that SCV catheters have a higher complication rate of clinically important thrombosis and stenosis than do IJV catheters used in hemodialysis and some oncology patients (28–33). Issues of venous stenosis secondary to SCV catheterization have not been as clearly demonstrated in other populations of patients. Central venous thrombosis secondary to indwelling catheters has been widely demonstrated in patient populations other than hemodialysis and oncology patients, but no study has compared the relative incidence of venous thrombosis between IJV and SCV catheterization in these populations. Another potential disadvantage of SCV catheter placement is the possibility of catheter pinch-off (34). This occurs when the catheter enters the SCV in an extravascular position between the first rib and clavicle, and the costoclavicular ligament and subclavius muscle impinge on the catheter. Entrapment at this location can cause repetitive stress on the catheter and can eventually result in catheter fracture and embolization. This complication can be avoided by a more lateral entry into the vein away from the junction of the clavicle and first rib.

Allowing for these considerations, the most commonly used venous access route today is the IJV. Studies have demonstrated this route to be very safe, with a high technical success rate and few procedural complications (35,36). Catheter placement via the IJV route has a comparable overall technical success to the SCV route, but with greater technical ease of accessing the vein under ultrasonographic guidance, thereby decreasing overall procedure time. This should be obvious when one considers the obscured location of the SCV beneath the clavicle as compared with the relatively superficial location of the IJV. In addition, the IJV approach has been shown to have a lower rate of procedure-related pneumothorax when compared with the SCV approach (37).

The right IJV approach is preferred over the left for practical reasons. The right IJV provides a straighter course to the right atrium; the left IJV route requires traversing the relatively acute angles at the left IJV-SCV and left brachiocephalic vein (BCV)-superior vena cava confluences. The resulting anatomic configuration on the left is more prone to catheter malposition, often resulting in the tip of the catheter tenting the lateral wall of the superior vena cava, a position that could potentially cause mediastinal perforation and massive hemorrhage. The left IJV tends to be smaller and deeper than the right IJV (38). Some studies have demonstrated that catheter patency rates are lower using the left-sided approach (39–42), but this might be due in part to the greater propensity for malposition on the left side, as discussed above.

Alternatives to the jugular and subclavian approaches often need to be considered when these routes have become thrombosed, as in patients requiring chronic central venous access. Among the alternatives are the femoral, translumbar, transhepatic, and azygous routes. Placement of an indwelling catheter via the femoral vein has the advantage of being technically easy, but it has been demonstrated that this route is associated with the need for more frequent interventions to maintain patency and a higher rate of infection than thoracic catheters (43). Translumbar cannulation of the inferior vena cava is essentially an extension of the translumbar aortography technique and has been in use since the mid 1980s, when Kenney et al. first reported on it (44). Transhepatic catheter placement, although an important alternative in a patient with no other viable access, should be limited to patients in whom translumbar catheters cannot be placed. This technique

requires percutaneous cannulation of a hepatic vein with placement of the catheter tip in the right atrium. Transhepatic catheters have all the risks and complications of tunneled catheters placed at other sites, in addition to the increased risks of significant bleeding (45) and hepatic vein occlusion with the potential sequela of acute Budd-Chiari syndrome (46). An additional disadvantage of this route is the effect of respiratory excursion on the liver, which could cause catheter dislodgement. The transhepatic route is also subject to the problems of any transhepatically placed catheter, which include bile leak, hepatic artery pseudoaneurysm, and patient discomfort. Alternate access routes are discussed in more detail in Chapter 12.

One of the great advantages of tunneled catheter placement by the interventional radiologist is the use of imaging guidance for gaining venous access. Prior to the advent of interventional radiology, access was gained either by surgical cutdown technique or blind percutaneous puncture. The minimally invasive nature of the percutaneous technique is its greatest advantage over the cutdown technique. Complications associated with blind percutaneous puncture range from 1% to 7% in the reported literature; these include pneumothorax, hemothorax, arteriovenous fistulae, and nerve injury (47,48). The reported rate of complication secondary to percutaneous puncture with imaging guidance is 0% to 2% (49,50).

For the IJV route, the patient is placed on the table with his or her head near the top of the table. This allows the operator to be comfortably positioned at the head of the table with the ultrasonography unit placed facing the operator; this positioning makes it easy for the operator to easily perform the puncture parallel to the course of the vein. Prior to preparing and draping the neck and chest, the operator should perform a brief ultrasonographic examination of the IJV to ascertain its patency (Fig. 7.3). Compressibility of the vein and lack of intraluminal echogenic thrombus are good indicators of patency. Central patency also can be evaluated by variation in vein caliber with respiratory motion; the vein decreases in size with inspiration and increases with expiration. If cyclical varia-

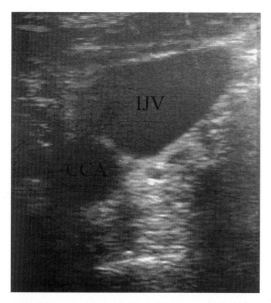

FIG. 7.3. Ultrasonographic image of the typical relationship between the common carotid artery (*CCA*) and the internal jugular vein (*IJV*).

tion in vein caliber is not demonstrated, a high-grade central stenosis or occlusion may be present and should be further evaluated. If the vein is of small caliber, it may be engorged by placing the patient's head down (reverse Trendelenburg position) if the angiography table is so equipped to tilt. Once the IJV patency is confirmed, the neck and chest are surgically prepared and draped from the angle of the mandible to the nipple line, and from the mid-axillary line to the sternum. Sterility of the ultrasonographic probe can be maintained with placement of a sterile cover. The skin overlying the venipuncture is anesthetized with 1% lidocaine; care should be taken to first flush the lidocaine through the 25-gauge anesthesia needle to avoid the injection of air into the subcutaneous tissue, because this could interfere with ultrasonographic visualization.

At our institution the venipuncture is performed with a 21-gauge micropuncture needle to minimize the risks of pneumothorax and inadvertent arterial puncture. A low IJV puncture site is preferred, which results in a smoother, more direct course for the catheter once it is brought through the subcutaneous tunnel; higher

punctures tend to result in a catheter course that assumes a sharper angle at the venous entry site and might contribute to catheter kinking and malfunction. The entry needle should be held at an angle parallel to the angle of the ultrasonographic transducer to assure visualization of the needle tip. If the probe is held at a more perpendicular angle to that of the needle, the tip of the needle can pass beyond the plane of visualization. This may result in a pneumothorax or arterial puncture because the common carotid artery or subclavian artery may be posterior to the IJV at the level of the clavicle. The needle is advanced under ultrasonographic guidance until it is seen indenting the anterior wall of the IJV. The needle is then jabbed through the vein wall; it is often helpful to ask the patient to perform a Valsalva maneuver at this time to help distend the vein. Once the needle has entered the vein, a 0.018-inch guidewire is advanced through the needle. If the access is venous, the course of the wire for a right IJV access should be relatively straight down the right lateral edge of the mediastinum and descend into the right atrium; the course of the wire from a left IJV approach should cross the mediastinum to the right of the spine and then descend to the right atrium. Deviation from these courses should alert the operator to the possibility of arterial puncture, which can be confirmed by the injection of a small amount of contrast through the needle. If the puncture is arterial, the needle and wire should be removed and compression held over the puncture site.

Attention is then turned to the creation of the subcutaneous tunnel (Figs. 7.4 and 7.5). The skin tunnel may be created either medially, to exit at a parasternal infraclavicular location, or laterally, to exit below the clavicle at the deltopectoral groove. A medial skin tunnel has the advantage of having less dependent chest wall weight pulling on the catheter and making catheter migration less likely, particularly in obese and large-breasted patients. It also may be more comfortable for women by keeping the catheter exit site away from bra straps. The advantage of a lateral skin tunnel is a more gently curved course that may be less prone to catheter kinking at the venotomy site. The decision for tun-

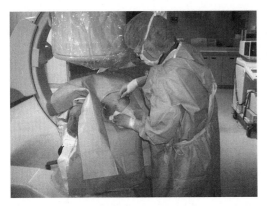

FIG. 7.4. The operator creates the subcutaneous tunnel by guiding the tunneler from the skin exit site at the deltopectoral groove toward the neck venotomy site.

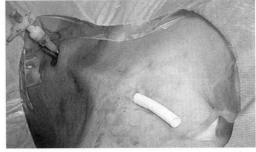

FIG. 7.5. Photograph demonstrating the placement of the skin tunneling device after it has been placed from the skin exit site and exteriorized at the venotomy site at the base of the neck. The distal tip of the catheter is then attached to the end of the tunneler at the skin exit site and pulled through the tunnel to exit at the venotomy site.

nel location should be made on a patient-by-patient basis depending on these individual factors.

The longer 21-gauge micropuncture needle used for access can be used to anesthetize the tract of subcutaneous tissue between the skin exit site and venotomy. The use of 2% lidocaine with epinephrine is helpful in limiting bleeding along the tunnel tract. A 1- to 2-cm skin incision is then made at the skin exit site; the incision length should approximate the diameter of the Dacron cuff to allow its passage. The tunnel is bluntly created by using a hemostat or, preferably, a commercially available tunneling device. A hemostat creates a wider than necessary tunnel, which results in unnecessary dead space; blood may pool in this extra subcutaneous space and contribute to future potential tunnel infections. The tunneling devices available are usually made of metal or plastic and have some degree of malleability, which allows the operator to steer the tunneler. Care is taken not to create the tunnel too superficially and cause puckering of the overlying skin, nor should it be so deep as to make retrieval of the cuff difficult when it is time to remove the catheter. The tunneler can be directed toward the venotomy by external manipulation with the operator's free hand and by applied countertraction on the overlying skin (Fig. 7.4). Once the tip is seen or felt at the venotomy incision, it

is exteriorized through the incision; this frequently requires sharp dissection to allow passage of the tunneler through the neck fascia (Fig. 7.5). Leaving the Dacron cuff within 1 to 2 cm of the skin exit site makes future removal of the catheter easier. In addition, when positioning the cuff within the tunnel (Fig. 7.6), it should

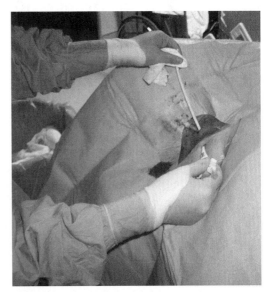

FIG. 7.6. The catheter position after it has been pulled through the subcutaneous tunnel as described in Fig. 7.5.

not be placed over the clavicle, which can be very uncomfortable for the patient and could cause pressure erosion and breakdowm of the overlying skin.

Other than for catheters intended for hemodialysis or apheresis, the catheter tip should be positioned at the cavoatrial junction. The catheter tip tends to migrate with changes in patient position; it tends to rest more caudally when the patient is in the supine position and rests significantly more cephalad in the upright position. The apparent change in catheter position is greater for catheters placed via the SCV route, and in females and obese patients, and is related to lower diaphragmatic excursion and the effects of the weight of the chest wall on the catheter when the patient is in the upright position (51).

Following the final dilatation, the peel-away sheath and its inner dilator are advanced over the guidewire. Advancement of the dilators and peel-away sheath should be performed under brief intermittent fluoroscopy to ascertain smooth passage over the guidewire. After the peel-away introducer sheath is placed, the patient is instructed to take a deep breath in, hold it, and perform a Valsalva maneuver while the guidewire and inner introducer are removed (Fig. 7.7). This is done to avoid air emboliza-

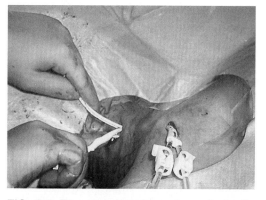

FIG. 7.8. The operator places the catheter tip through the peel-away sheath. The catheter is secured in place with the tip of the index finger while the sheath is peeled away.

tion through the sheath if the patient should inspire while the operator is in the process of placing the tip of the catheter into the sheath. Another preventive measure is to pull the sheath back a few centimeters and pinch it at the skin after the inner dilator and guidewire have been pulled out. The catheter is then quickly advanced through the sheath and the patient given instruction to breathe normally once again (Fig. 7.8). After peel-away sheath removal, the catheter position is evaluated under fluoroscopy; the course of the catheter also should be examined to assure there are no kinks in the catheter that would obstruct flow. If a kink in the catheter is demonstrated, passage of a stiff glide hydrophilic wire through the lumen often helps to smooth out the course and to eliminate the kink in the catheter.

The venotomy site is closed with a single subcuticular stitch of absorbable suture material. A nonabsorbable monofilament suture is placed at the skin exit site and secured around the catheter. Dry sterile dressings are then placed at the venotomy and skin exit sites. Each catheter port is filled with heparin solution at a concentration of 100 U/mL.

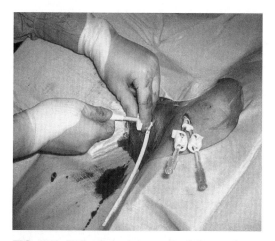

FIG. 7.7. Following placement of the catheter through the subcutaneous tunnel, the operator removes the inner dilator of the peel-away sheath in preparation for intravascular placement of the catheter.

POSTPROCEDURAL CONSIDERATIONS

Following routine IJV or SCV catheter placement, it is not necessary to obtain a chest radiograph if the venous access procedure was performed under imaging guidance and the catheter position confirmed under fluoroscopy. Several recent studies suggest this algorithm (52–54). The largest study to date was a prospective study of 937 consecutive central venous catheter placements, including ports, tunneled, and nontunneled catheters. No postprocedure chest radiograph demonstrated a complication that was not already apparent during the procedure, and only one malpositioned catheter that required further manipulation was found in the series (53). In addition, the charges associated with obtaining the films added significantly to the cost of the procedure as well as unnecessarily increasing the procedure-related nursing time by an average of 23 minutes (53).

At our institution, following the procedure patients are taken to a postanesthesia recovery area for monitoring for 1 to 2 hours prior to discharge, or return back to their room. Prior to discharge, nursing instructions are given to the patient, which include education as to the signs of catheter-related infection and routine catheter care. If patients are unable to perform routine catheter care, arrangements are made for visiting nurse care.

Routine catheter care includes daily irrigation of the catheter to prevent occlusion secondary to thrombosis or medication precipitation within the lumen of the catheter. Hickman and Broviac type catheters should be flushed twice a day and after each use with saline or heparinized saline at a concentration of 100 U/mL. Groshong-type catheters are flushed once a week and after each use with saline. Also important are routine dressing changes, which have been demonstrated to decrease catheter infection rates (55–57). Gauze and tape or breathable transparent dressings are recommended on the first day after catheter placement and then three times a week. For neutropenic or otherwise immunocompromised patients, consideration should be given to daily dressing changes. The dressing at the venotomy site can be removed after the first 24 hours. Postprocedural care guidelines are dis-

cussed more fully in Chapter 10 (Ray and Paplham).

COMPLICATIONS

Complications of central venous access are more fully discussed in Chapter 14, but a brief review is offered here with special attention to those complications specifically related to tunneled catheters. Complications can be grouped into two broad categories: early (or periprocedural) and late. Early complications are those that occur at the time of catheter placement, whereas late complications are those not necessarily related to catheter placement and occur following insertion. Early complications include failure to gain venous access, pneumothorax, inadvertent arterial puncture, air embolus, nerve damage, catheter malposition and malfunction, arrhythmias, and great vessel perforation. Late complications include infections, thrombosis, delayed catheter migration, and catheter fracture and embolization. The two most common indications for early tunneled catheter removal are catheter-related venous thrombosis and catheter infection; these are more fully addressed here as they relate to tunneled catheters.

Thrombotic events occurring as a complication of Hickman and Broviac catheters range from fibrin sheath formation around the catheter tip to major central venous thrombosis. Fibrin sheaths have been estimated to form in 42% to 100% of patients with indwelling catheters (58–60). They interfere with catheter function by either occluding the lumen or by acting as a one-way valve; a typical history suggestive of a fibrin sheath is that the catheter flushes easily, but blood cannot be aspirated from the port. The diagnosis can be confirmed by contrast injection through the catheter, which could demonstrate filling defects around the catheter tip, occlusion of flow at the distal tip of the catheter, or backflow of contrast along the side of the catheter within the fibrin sheath. Catheter malfunction secondary to fibrin sheath formation can be managed by exchanging the catheter, mechanically stripping the fibrin sheath from around the catheter, or infusing tissue plasminogen activator (TPA) through the catheter. If the catheter is exchanged over a wire without addressing the underlying problem of the fibrin sheath, the new catheter may slip into the sheath with the same catheter malfunction. To avoid this possibility, a gentle venous angioplasty along the catheter course can be performed to disrupt the fibrin sheath prior to placement of the new catheter (61,62). Another described therapy is to strip the catheter with a wire snare advanced from the common femoral vein (63). The least invasive, yet still effective, option is the instillation of a thrombolytic agent to dwell within the catheter lumen or infusion of the thrombolytic through the catheter lumen over a few hour period (64). Since the thrombolytic urokinase was removed from the market, its void has been filled by TPA. At our institution, fibrin sheaths are initially treated by placing TPA, at a concentration of 1 mg/mL, in each lumen to dwell within and to fill the lumen. If catheter malfunction persists, a short-term infusion of TPA is administered. Each lumen of the catheter is treated with 2 mg of TPA diluted to a volume of 50 mL and infused into the catheter over a 4-hour period.

Of the above-mentioned options, it is preferable to salvage the catheter rather than exchange it for a new one, unless there is an infectious or other complication that requires catheter removal. The technique of catheter stripping with a snare was described by Haskal et al. for hemodialysis catheters, but the study only demonstrated initial success of the technique without durable benefit (65). A more recent and larger patient population study by Brady et al. showed a median primary patency of 3 months following hemodialysis catheter stripping (66). Although catheter stripping demonstrated reasonable results in this series, it is probably more cost efficient to treat a fibrin sheath with TPA, either by injecting the catheter and allowing the TPA to dwell within the lumen or to perform a short-term infusion through the catheter as discussed above.

At the other end of the range of thrombotic complications of indwelling catheters is major central venous thrombosis, which has been reported in 3% to 17% of patients with Hickman and Broviac catheters (67). Central venous thrombosis often occurs without symptoms, but upper extremity edema and superior vena cava syndrome have been described (68). Several factors have been identified that increase the risk for central thrombosis, which include left-sided approach, subclavian vein approach, positioning of the catheter tip within the proximal superior vena cava or brachiocephalic vein, underlying malignancy, and more than one indwelling catheter (69–73). Low-dose coumadin therapy (1 mg/day) has been shown to decrease the incidence of catheter-related central venous thrombosis in oncology patients with chest ports (74) and may be beneficial in patients with tunneled catheters with one or more of the above-mentioned risk factors (75).

The incidence of Hickman and Broviac catheter infections is reported between 15% and 20% in the literature (76,77) and can be categorized into skin tract infections, catheter-related sepsis, and catheter-related septic thrombophlebitis. Skin tract infections can be further subdivided into exit site infections if involvement is within 2 cm of the skin exit site, and tunnel infections if involvement extends beyond 2 cm of the skin exit site. Catheter-related sepsis is defined as fever and bacteremia without skin tract infection, in addition to quantitative blood cultures demonstrating a tenfold greater colony count in samples obtained through the catheter as compared with peripherally obtained blood cultures. In a series by Press et al., exit site infections accounted for 45.5% of tunneled catheter infections, bacteremia/septicemia accounted for 30.8%, tunnel infections accounted for 20.3%, and septic thrombophlebitis accounted for 3.5% (78). The most common organisms in the same series were *Staphylococcus epidermidis* (54%) and *Staphylococcus aureus* (20%). Less common organisms included *Candida albicans* (5.9%), *Pseudomonas* species (5.9%), and diphtheroids (4.7%) (78).

The pathogenesis of catheter-related infections is complex, with several potential sources of contamination. There is strong evidence for the migration of skin flora along the subcutaneous tunnel, with eventual colonization of the catheter tip (79–82). There are also significant data to support the theory that contamination of the catheter hub can result in intraluminal colonization of the catheter (83–85). There has been much debate as to which of these mechanisms has greater impact on the development of catheter-related infections. Some data suggest that the length of time of catheterization in part determines which of the processes predominates. For catheters in place for over 1 month, hub contamination appears to play the major role; for catheters in place for less than 10 days, skin contamination is the more probable mechanism (86). Other mechanisms also have a role in the development of catheter infections, but much less commonly than the aforementioned mechanisms. Among these are hematogenous seeding of the catheter from a distant focus of infection and administration of infected infusate through the catheter (85,87–88).

The management of infectious complications of tunneled catheters depends on the category of catheter infection. Exit site infections can be treated with local wound care and antibiotics; usually the catheter does not have to be removed. Most tunnel infections are caused by coagulase-negative staphylococci and are initially treated with intravenous vancomycin (89). In cases of exit and tunnel infections that do not respond to treatment within 48 hours, catheter removal is recommended (89). It should be noted that most tunnel infections do not respond to therapy and require catheter removal (89). Catheter-related sepsis mandates catheter removal and treatment with the appropriate antibiotics, as indicated by blood culture and sensitivities. Septic thrombophlebitis is also an indication for catheter removal and treatment with appropriate antibiotic coverage and anticoagulation.

REFERENCES

1. Thomas JH, MacArthur RI, Pierce GE, et al. Hickman-Broviac catheters: indications and results. *Am J Surg* 1980;140:791–796.

2. Broviac JW, Cole JJ, Scribner BH. A silicone rubber atrial catheter for prolonged parenteral alimentation. *Surg Gynecol Obstet* 1973;136:602–606.

3. Ponsky JL, Gauderer WL. Expanded applications of Broviac catheter. *Arch Surg* 1980;115:324.

4. Bozzetti F, Scarpa D, Terno G, et al. Subclavian venous thrombosis due to indwelling catheters: a prospective study on 52 patients. *J Parenter Enter Nutr* 1983;7:560–562.

5. Flowers RH, Schwenzer KJ, Kopel RF, et al. Efficacy of an attachable subcutaneous cuff for the prevention of intravascular catheter-related infection. *JAMA* 1989;261:878–883.

6. Maki DG, Cobb L, Garman JK, et al. An attachable silver-impregnated cuff for prevention of infection with central venous catheters: a prospective randomized multicenter trial. *Am J Med* 1988;85:307–314.

7. Dahlberger PJ, Agger WA, Singer JR, et al. Subclavian hemodialysis catheterinfections: randomized trial of an attachable silver-impregnated cuff for the prevention of catheter-related infections. *Infect Control Hosp Epidemiol* 1995;16:506–511.

8. Babycos CR, Barrocos A, Webb WR. A prospective randomized trial comparing the silver-impregnated collagen cuff with the bedside tunneled subclavian catheter. *J Parenter Enter Nutr* 1993; 17:61–63.

9. Groeger JS, Lucas AB, Coit D, et al. A prospective randomized evaluation of the effect of silver-impregnated subcutaneous cuffs for preventing tunneled chronic venous access catheter infections in cancer patients. *Ann Surg* 1993;218:206–210.

10. Hemmerlein JB, Trerotola SO, Kraus MA, et al. *In vitro* cytotoxicity of silver-impregnated collagen cuffs designed to decrease infection in tunneled catheters. *Radiology* 1997;204:363–367.

11. Robertson LJ, Mauro MA, Jaques PF. Radiologic placement of Hickman catheters. *Radiology* 1989;170:1007–1009.

12. Lameris JS, Post PJM, Zonderland HM, et al. Percutaneous placement of Hickman catheters: comparison of sonographically guided and blind techniques. *AJR* 1990;155:1097–1099.

13. Hanks SE, Pentecost M, Katz MD, et al. Cost savings with radiologic versus surgical placement of central venous access catheters. *Radiology* 1992;185:322.

14. Mauro MA, Jaques PF. Radiologic placement of long term central venous access catheters: a review. *J Vasc Intervent Radiol* 1993;4:127–137.

15. Docktor BL, Sadler DJ, Gray RR et al. Radiologic placement of tunneled central catheters: rates of success and of immediate complications in a large series. *AJR* 1999;173:457–460.

16. Warner BW, Haygood MM, Davies SL, et al. A randomized prospective trial of standard Hickman compared with Groshong central venous catheters in pediatric oncology patients. *J Am Coll Surg* 1996;183:140–144.

17. Pasquale MD, Campbell JM, Magnant CM. Groshong versus Hickman catheters. *Surg Gynecol Obstet* 1992; 174:408–410.

18. Dearborn P, DeMuth JS, Requarth AB, et al. Nurse and patient satisfaction with three types of venous access devices. *Oncol Nurs Forum* 1997;24(suppl):34–40.

19. Keung YK, Watkins K, Chen SC, et al. Comparative study of infectious complications of different types of

chronic central venous access devices. *Cancer* 1994; 73:2832–2837.

20. Ranson MR, Oppenheim BA, Jackson A, et al. Double-blind placebo controlled study of vancomycin prophylaxis for central venous catheter insertion in cancer patients. *J Hosp Infect* 1990;15:95–102.

21. McKee R, Dunsmuir R, Whitby M, et al. Does antibiotic prophylaxis at the time of catheter insertion reduce the incidence of catheter-related sepsis in intravenous nutrition? *J Hosp Infect* 1985;6:419–425.

22. Dravid VS, Gupta A, Zegel HG, et al. Investigation of antibiotic prophylaxis usage for vascular and nonvascular interventional procedures. *J Vasc Intervent Radiol* 1998;9:401–406.

23. Mauro MA, Jaques PF. Radiologic placement of long-term central venous catheters: a review. *J Vasc Intervent Radiol* 1993;4:127–137.

24. Denny DR, Jr. The role of the radiologist in long-term central vein access. *Radiology* 1992;185:637–638.

25. Sabatelli FW, Hawkins IF, Kerns SR. Radiologic versus surgical placement of long-term indwelling central venous access catheters: a retrospective review [Abstract]. *Radiology* 1993;189:199.

26. Hull JE, Hunter CS, Luiken GA. The Groshong catheter: initial experience and early results of image-guided placement. *Radiology* 1992;185:803–807.

27. Morris SL, Jaques PF, Mauro MA. Radiology-assisted placement of implantable subcutaneous infusion ports for long-term venous access. *Radiology* 1992;184: 149–151.

28. Beenan L, van Leusen R, Deenik B, et al. The incidence of subclavian vein stenosis using silicone catheters for hemodialysis. *Artif Organs* 1994;18:289–292.

29. Cimochowski GE, Worley E, Rutherford WE, et al. Superiority of the internal jugular over the subclavian access for temporary dialysis. *Nephron* 1990;54: 154–161.

30. Spinowitz BS, Galler M, Golden RA, et al. Subclavian vein stenosis as a complication of subclavian catheterization for hemodialysis. *Arch Intern Med* 1987;147: 303–307.

31. Vanherweghem JL, Yassine T, Goldman M, et al. Subclavian vein thrombosis: a frequent complication of subclavian vein cannulation for hemodialysis. *Clin Nephrol* 1986;26:235–238.

32. DeMoor B, Vanholder R, Ringoir S. Subclavian vein hemodialysis catheters: advantages and disadvantages. *Artif Organs* 1994;18:293–297.

33. Schwab SJ, Quarles D, Middleton JP, et al. Hemodialysis associated subclavian vein stenosis. *Kidney Int* 1988;33:1156–1159.

34. Hinke DH, Zandt-Stanley DA, Goodman LR, et al. Pinch-off syndrome: a complication of implanted subclavian venous access devices. *Radiology* 1990;177: 353–356.

35. Trerotola SO, Johnson MS, Harris VJ, et al. Outcome of tunneled hemodialysis catheters placed via the right internal jugular vein by interventional radiologists. *Radiology* 1997;203:489–495.

36. Silberzweig JE, Mitty HA. Central venous access: low internal jugular vein approach using imaging guidance. *AJR* 1998;170:1617–1620.

37. Macdonald S, Watt AJ, McNally D, et al. Comparison of technical success and outcome of tunneled catheters inserted via the jugular and subclavian approaches. *J Vasc Intervent Radiol* 2000;11(part 1):225–231.

38. Gordon AC, Saliken JC, Johns D, et al. Ultrasound-guided puncture of the internal jugular vein: complications and anatomic considerations. *J Vasc Intervent Radiol* 1998;9:333–338.

39. Surratt RS, Picus D, Hicks ME, et al. The importance of preoperative evaluation of the subclavian vein in dialysis access planning. *AJR* 1991;156:623–625.

40. De Meester J, Vanholder R, Ringoir S. Factors affecting catheter and technique survival in permanent silicone single-lumen dialysis catheters [Abstract]. *Nephrol Dial Transplant* 1994;9:678–683.

41. Glanz S, Gordon D, Lipkowitz G, et al. Axillary and subclavian vein stenosis: percutaneous angioplasty. *Radiology* 1988;168:371–373.

42. Puel V, Caudry M, Le Metayer P, et al. Superior vena cava thrombosis relative to catheter malposition in cancer chemotherapy given through implanted ports. *Cancer* 1993;72:2248–2252.

43. Zaleski GX, Funaki B, Lorenz JM, et al. Experience with tunneled femoral hemodialysis catheters. *AJR* 1999;172:493–496.

44. Kenney PR, Dorfman GS, Denny DF Jr. Percutaneous inferior vena cava cannulation for long term parenteral nutrition. *Surgery* 1985;97:602–605.

45. Putnam SG, Ball D, Cohen GS. Transhepatic dialysis catheter tract embolization to close a venous-biliary-peritoneal fistula. *J Vasc Intervent Radiol* 1998;9:149–151.

46. Pieters PC, Dittrich J, Prasad U, et al. Acute Budd-Chiari syndrome caused by percutaneous placement of a transhepatic IVC catheter. *J Vasc Intervent Radiol* 1997;8:587–590.

47. Davis SJ, Thompson JS, Edney JA. Insertion of Hickman catheters: a comparison of cutdown and percutaneous techniques. *Am Surg* 1984;50:673–676.

48. Ryan JA, Abel RM, Abbott WM, et al. Catheter complications in total parenteral nutrition. *N Engl J Med* 1974;290:757–761.

49. Lameris JS, Post PJM, Zonderland HM, et al. Percutaneous placement of Hickman catheters: comparison of sonographically guided and blind techniques. *AJR* 1990;155:1097–1099.

50. Mallory DL, McGee WT, Shawker TH, et al. Ultrasound guidance improves the success rate of internal jugular vein cannulation. *Chest* 1990;98:157–160.

51. Nazarian GK, Bjarnson H, Dietz CA, et al.Changes in tunneled catheter tip position when a patient is upright. *J Vasc Intervent Radiol* 1997;8:437–441.

52. Chang TC, Funaki B, Szymski GX. Are routine chest radiographs necessary after image-guided placement of internal jugular central venous access devices? *AJR* 1998;170:335–337.

53. Caridi JG, West JH, Stavropoulos SW, et al. Internal jugular and upper extremity central vein access in interventional radiology: is a post procedure x-ray necessary? *AJR* 2000;174:363–366.

54. Lucey B, Varghese JC, Haslan P, et al. Routine chest radiographs after central line insertion: mandatory post procedural evaluation or unnecessary waste of resources? *Cardiovasc Intervent Radic!* 1999;22:381–384.

55. Jones GR. A practical guide to evaluation and treatment of infections in patients with central venous catheters. *J Intraven Nurs* 1998;21(suppl):134–142.

56. Sheretz RJ. Surveillance for infections associated with vascular catheters. *Infect Control Hosp Epidemiol* 1996;17:746–752.

57. La Voie K, Kopnick M. Impact of dressing materials on central venous catheter infection rates. *J Intraven Nurs* 1998;21:140–142.

58. Brisman B, Hardstedt C, Jacobson S. Diagnosis of thrombosis by catheter phlebography after prolonged central venous catheterization. *Ann Surg* 1981;194:779–783.

59. Peters WR, Bush WH, McIntyre RD, et al. The development of fibrin sheath on indwelling venous catheters. *Surg Gynecol Obstet* 1973;137:43–47.

60. Raad I, Luna M, Khalil SAM, et al. The relationship between the thrombotic and infectious complications of central venous catheters. *JAMA* 1994;271:1014–1016.

61. Suhocki PV, Conlon PJ, Knelson MH, et al. Silicone cuffed catheters for hemodialysis vascular access: thrombolytic and mechanical correction of malfunction. *Am J Kidney Dis* 1996;28:379–386.

62. Brown PWG, McBride KD, Gaines PA. Technical report: Hickman catheter rescue. *Clin Radiol* 1994;49:891–894.

63. Crain MR, Mewissen MW, Ostrowski GJ, et al. Fibrin sleeve stripping for salvage of failing hemodialysis catheters: technique and initial results. *Radiology* 1996;198:41–44.

64. Haire WD, Lieberman RP, Lund GB, et al. Obstructed central venous catheters. *Cancer* 1990;66:2279–2285.

65. Haskal ZJ, Leen VH, Thomas Hawkins C, et al. Transvenous removal of fibrin sheath from tunneled hemodialysis catheters. *J Vasc Intervent Radiol* 1996;7:513–517.

66. Brady PS, Spence LD, Levitin A, et al. Efficacy of percutaneous fibrin sheath stripping in restoring patency of tunneled hemodialysis catheters. *AJR* 1999;173:1023–1027.

67. Fan CM. Tunneled catheters. *Semin Intervent Radiol* 1998;15:273–286.

68. Kerr HD. Superior vena cava syndrome associated with a Hickman catheter. *NY State J Med* 1990;April:208–209.

69. Haire WD, Lieberman RP, Edney J, et al. Hickman catheter induced thoracic vein thrombosis. *Cancer* 1990;66:900–908.

70. Anderson AJ, Krasnow SH, Boyer MW, et al. Thrombosis: the major Hickman catheter complication in patients with solid tumor. *Chest* 1989;95:71–75.

71. Moss JF, Wagman LD, Riihimaki DU, et al. Central venous thrombosis related to the silastic Hickman-Broviac catheter in oncologic patients. *J Parenter Enter Nutr* 1989;13:397–400.

72. Eastridge BJ, Lefor AT. Complications of indwelling venous access devices in cancer patients. *J Clin Oncol* 1995;13:233–238.

73. Craft PS, May J, Hoy C, et al. Hickman catheters: left-sided insertion, male gender, and obesity are associated with an increased risk of complications. *Aust NZ J Med* 1996;26:33–39.

74. Boraks P, Seale J, Price J, et al. Prevention of central venous catheter associated thrombosis using minidose warfarin in patients with haematological malignancies. *Br J Haematol* 1998;101:483–486.

75. Bern MM, Lokich JJ, Wallach SR, et al. Very low doses of warfarin can prevent thrombosis in central venous catheters. *Ann Intern Med* 1990;112:423–428.

76. Clark DE, Raffin TA. Infectious complications of indwelling long-term central venous catheters. *Chest* 1990;97:966–972.

77. Johnson A, Oppenheim BA. Vascular catheter-related sepsis: diagnosis and prevention. *J Hosp Infect* 1992;20:67–78.

78. Press OW, Ramsey PG, Larson EB, et al. Hickman catheter infections in patients with malignancies. *Medicine* 1984;63:189–200.

79. Bjarnson HS, Colley R, Bower RH, et al. Association between microorganism growth at the catheter insertion site and colonization of the catheter in patients receiving total parenteral nutrition. *Surgery* 1982;92:720–727.

80. Cooper GL, Hopkins CC. Rapid diagnosis of intravascular catheter-associated infection by direct gram staining of catheter segments. *N Engl J Med* 1985;312:1142–1147.

81. Kelsey MC, Gosling M. A comparison of the morbidity associated with occlusive and nonocclusive dressings applied to peripheral intravenous devices. *J Hosp Infect* 1984;5:313–321.

82. Snydman DR, Pober BR, Murray SA, et al. Predictive value of surveillance skin cultures in total peripheral nutrition-related infection. Prospective epidemiologic study using semi quantitative cultures. *Lancet* 1982;2:1385–1388.

83. deCicco M, Chiaradia V, Veronesi A, et al. Source and route of microbial colonization of parenteral nutrition catheters. *Lancet* 1989;2:1258–1261.

84. Salzman MB, Isenberg HD, Shapiro JF, et al. A prospective study of the catheter hub as the portal of entry for microorganisms causing catheter related sepsis in neonates. *J Infect Dis* 1993;167:487–490.

85. Linares J, Sitges-Serra A, Garau J, et al. Pathogenesis of catheter sepsis: a prospective study with quantitative and semi quantitative cultures of catheter hub and segments. *J Clin Microbiol* 1985;21:357–360.

86. Raad I, Costerton W, Sabharwal U, et al. Ultrastructural analysis of indwelling vascular catheters: a quantitative relationship between lumenal colonization and duration of placement. *J Infect Dis* 1993;168:400–407.

87. Maki DG, Martin WT. Nationwide epidemic of septicemia caused by contaminated infusion products. IV: Growth of microbial pathogens in fluids for intravenous injection. *J Infect Dis* 1975;131:267–272.

88. Centers for Disease Control. Nosocomial bacteremia associated with intravenous fluid therapy. *MMWR* 1971;20(suppl 9):81–82.

89. Pearson ML. Guideline for prevention of intravascular-device-related infections. *Infect Control Hosp Epidemiol* 1996;17:438–473.

Central Venous Access
Edited by Charles E. Ray, Jr.
Lippincott Williams & Wilkins, Philadelphia © 2001.

8

Hemodialysis Access

James H. Turner, MD

Department of Radiology, Denver Health Medical Center;
University of Colorado Health Sciences Center, Denver, Colorado 80209

In the United States alone, there are approximately 300,000 patients with end-stage renal disease (ESRD). Treatment options for ESRD include renal transplantation, peritoneal dialysis, and hemodialysis, with approximately 62% of all patients maintained on chronic hemodialysis. Hemodialysis requires access to the circulatory system on a chronic, intermittent basis. Access is achieved by two primary means, namely surgically created arteriovenous shunts and dialysis catheters. A surgical shunt is created in an extremity, by formation of an arteriovenous fistula (AVF) or placement of a synthetic graft. An AVF is created by connecting a native vein to a native artery, usually in an end-to-side or side-to-side fashion. In contrast, a synthetic bridge graft, typically made of polytetrafluoroethylene, is placed from artery to vein. Advantages to AVFs are that they have a longer primary patency rate compared with grafts (1), but fistulas must be allowed to mature for months prior to use. Grafts, by contrast, can be used almost immediately. Whether an AVF or graft is used, shunts represent the most established form of dialysis access, and are the preferred form of long-term dialysis access because of their relatively long service lives and their lower rate of complications relative to catheters (2).

Surgical shunts and catheters have advantages and disadvantages relative to each other. First, in most cases shunts take weeks or months to mature before they can be used; conversely, patients can dialyze immediately after placement of a catheter. Second, hemodialysis catheters are more easily placed than surgical shunts. In an established venous access practice, a patient can usually be scheduled for catheter placement the same or the next day, and emergent hemodialysis can be performed in a patient with no access by placing a temporary central catheter. In contrast, surgical shunts require operating room time, anesthesia coverage, and a vascular surgeon proficient in dialysis access, each of which might not always be immediately available.

The mean patency of a synthetic surgical shunt is approximately 20 months, whereas native AVFs remain patent on average for 34 months (3). Whether an AVF or graft, surgical shunts fail for one main reason. By increasing the blood flow through a normal vein, as occurs through the venous side of a shunt, the endothelium is damaged and proliferates, eventually leading to stricture and occlusion. Pathologically this endothelial proliferation is termed neointimal hyperplasia. Angiographically, in grafts neointimal hyperplasia is visualized as focal tapered narrowing at the graft anastomosis site (Fig. 8.1). Although other factors such as arterial anastomotic strictures in grafts or narrowing of the fistula itself in AVFs may occur, in addition to distal venous outflow stenoses, the majority of grafts occlude secondary to stenoses at the venous anastomosis.

Once shunt failure occurs, access must be reestablished by surgical revision or radiologic intervention of the existing shunt. If these methods fail, the creation of a new shunt may be required. In the interim, dialysis is still re-

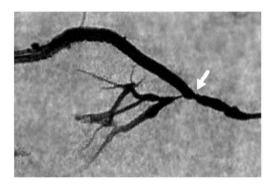

FIG. 8.1. Fistulogram demonstrating neointimal hyperplasia resulting in stenosis (arrow) at the venous anastomosis of a loop-graft.

quired and venous access must be maintained. Catheters, therefore, are commonly used as a bridge for hemodialysis, providing access until the more permanent surgical shunt can be established and allowed to mature. Hemodialysis catheters suffer from complications that limit their life span, however, including thrombosis, fibrin sheath formation, and infection. Treatment of catheter complications, which are discussed below, extends their useful life, but not enough to replace surgical shunts as a means of obtaining primary access. In patients who have had multiple shunt failures and have no peripheral veins left with which to create a new shunt, catheters become the primary means of maintaining circulatory access. Once a patient becomes obligated to catheter hemodialysis, their long-term prognosis worsens appreciably as evidenced by a marked increase in their mortality rate. All efforts are made, therefore, to reestablish a surgical shunt.

EVOLUTION OF
THE HEMODIALYSIS CATHETER

The use of a silicone rubber catheter for prolonged venous access was first described in 1973 (4). As described in this sentinel article, the catheter was tunneled subcutaneously and had a Dacron cuff to help retain the catheter in place; these two features have been retained to the current day. As well as acting as an anchor

to hold the catheter in place, the Dacron cuff helps prevent infection by eliciting growth of fibroblasts around the cuff. This fibrotic reaction forms a physical barrier to bacteria, preventing the skin exit site from becoming a portal for bacterial migration and inoculation. In 1979, Hickman et al. made improvements by increasing the size of the internal lumen of the catheter from 0.22 mm to 0.32 mm (5).

As opposed to venous access for parenteral nutrition or chemotherapy, hemodialysis requires flow of blood out of the body, through the dialysate, and back into the vascular system via separate channels. A dual-lumen catheter was first described for the purpose of dialysis in 1988 (6). There is an arterial port, which carries blood from the body, and a venous port, which returns blood to the venous system. The distal tips of the catheter are staggered to decrease mixing (recirculation) of blood. The initial tunneled catheter, which was commonly used for hemodialysis, was the Perm-Cath (Quinton Instrument Company, Seattle, WA, U.S.A.), which has subsequently become a common moniker for all cuffed, tunneled hemodialysis catheters.

Hemodialysis catheters continue to evolve. Increased lumen diameter has been the trend in catheter design, because increased lumen diameter means increased flow rates. Increasing the catheter flow rates allows faster dialysis, thereby decreasing the amount of time a patient must be attached to the dialysis machine (and increasing the number of patients who can undergo dialysis on any given day). The initial PermCaths, with an internal lumen diameter of 2 mm, achieved flow rates of 200 mL/min (6). Modern dialysis machines, however, can achieve effective dialysis at flow rates as high as 500 mL/min. The Tesio twin catheter was designed to accommodate increased flow rates, but this system is constructed as two completely separate catheters (7–9). The most recent catheter designs achieve flow rates comparable with that of the Tesio system but have the advantage of being a single-piece design (10,11). Catheter comparisons are made below.

CHOICE OF VENOTOMY SITE

Access sites for catheter insertion include the internal jugular veins, the axillary or subclavian veins, the common femoral veins, and the inferior vena cava. Insertion into the subclavian veins is associated with a high rate of venous stricture formation and occlusion at the catheter site (12,13). The purported mechanism of stricture formation is mechanical friction of the catheter against the vein endothelium as the vein crosses the first rib. In addition, transmitted cardiac pulsations through the catheter may provide a second source of mechanical friction.

Using the upper extremities for shunt placement makes preserving the integrity of the subclavian veins important. As stated previously, the altered hemodynamics associated with hemodialysis shunts can, by itself, lead to venous strictures. Causing damage to the subclavian veins with subsequent narrowing following catheter insertions must be avoided in order to preserve venous outflow from the upper extremities.

For the reasons presented above, the right internal jugular vein is the preferred insertion site. If the right internal jugular vein is occluded, the second choice for insertion site has not been firmly established in the literature. Many practicing interventional radiologists consider the left internal jugular vein the next best choice, because the femoral veins are an inconvenience for the patient while on outpatient dialysis. A translumbar catheter placed directly into the inferior vena cava is reserved for patients with no other access.

CHOICE OF CATHETER

Many hemodialysis catheters are commercially available (Fig. 8.2). As stated earlier, the trend in catheter design has been toward larger-diameter lumens to accommodate higher flow rates. Most catheters are of a single piece design with two separate lumens. The exception is the Tesio twin catheter (Medcomp, Harleysville, PA, U.S.A.), composed of two separate, single-lumen catheters. Each single-lumen cath-

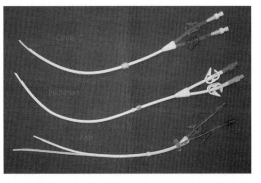

FIG. 8.2. Photograph of the various catheter types.

eter is placed in its own subcutaneous tunnel with its own venotomy. The single-piece, dual lumen catheters include Opti-Flow, Hickman, and Soft-Cell (Bard Access Systems, Salt Lake City, UT, U.S.A.); Schon Cath (Angiodynamics, Queensbury, NY, U.S.A.); Ash (Medcomp); Neostar Circle C (Horizon Medical Products, Manchester, GA, U.S.A.); and PermCath (Quinton Instrument Company, Seattle, WA, U.S.A.). The profiles of the single-piece catheters are different (round vs. oval outer catheter, split vs. nonsplit tips, two separate subcutaneous tunnels vs. one, etc.), with each catheter design possessing individual benefits and drawbacks. Table 8.1 lists the characteristics of each catheter.

Brief mention should be made of acute dialysis catheters. These catheters are for short-term access, most frequently within the hospital setting. The catheters are placed directly into the venotomy site without creating a subcutaneous tunnel. They are usually fashioned from polyurethane, giving them greater stiffness to allow the catheters to be placed directly over a wire rather than by using a peel-away sheath. The acute catheters do not have a Dacron cuff, and typically have smaller lumens than the cuffed, tunneled variety. All of the aforementioned manufacturers produce acute dialysis catheters as well as tunneled catheters.

Unlike tunneled catheters, acute care catheters do not require a full surgical preparation;

TABLE 8.1. *Commonly used tunneled hemodialysis catheters*

	Manufacturer	Material	Catheter size	Introducer	Lumen config/ tip config
Circle C	HMP, Manchester, GA	Silicone	13.5 Fr	14 Fr	Round/ staggered
Opti-Flow	Bard, Salt Lake City, UT	Polyurethane	14.5 Fr	15 Fr	Ds/staggered
Hickman	Bard	Silicone	13.5 Fr	14 Fr	Ds/staggered
Soft-Cell	Bard	Polyurethane	12.5 Fr	13 Fr	Ds/staggered
Ash	Medcomp, Harleysville, PA	Polyurethane	14 Fr	16 Fr	Round/split
Schon Cath	Angiodynamic, Queensbury, NY	Silicone	?	18 Fr	Round/split
Tesio	Medcomp	Silicone	10 Fr	11 Fr	Round, two separate venotomies
PermCath	Quinton, Seattle, WA	Silicone	12.5 Fr	18 Fr	Round/ staggered

standard angiographic sterile technique is adequate. Most catheters are commercially available in a kit form in which all necessary materials are included. Using a microaccess kit (Cook, Inc., Bloomington, IN, U.S.A.) may decrease the risk of insertion-related complications. As is the case with tunneled catheters, acute dialysis catheters should only be placed in the internal jugular veins in order to decrease the risk of catheter-related central venous stenosis.

TECHNIQUE FOR INSERTION

All of the commercially available hemodialysis catheters are available in kit form. The kits supply all the necessary items to place the catheters using variations of the Seldinger technique. Depending on the experience and preference of the operator, some of the items in the kit may be exchanged; for instance, the operator may not like the wire provided with the catheter kit and use an extra stiff or hydrophilic wire instead. Many operators prefer to use a micropuncture kit (Cook) to obtain initial access rather than the needles and wires provided in the kits.

General concepts related to placement of venous access devices (VADs) are presented in detail in Chapter 3. The remainder of this section briefly discusses general VAD placement techniques, specifically with regard to hemodialysis catheter placement.

An ultrasonographic examination is initially performed to confirm patency of the vein. Multiple investigators have demonstrated that direct visualization of the vein with ultrasonography reduces complications (14–16). Following ultrasonographic interrogation, the insertion site is prepared in sterile fashion. At our institution, the skin is cleansed first with Hibiclens (ICI Americas Inc, Wilmington, DE, U.S.A.), followed by a scrub with Betadine solution (Purdue Frederick Co., Norwalk, CT, U.S.A.). A large sterile drape is placed over the entire patient, with a fenestration over the catheter insertion and exit sites. Following administration of local anesthesia and under direct ultrasonographic guidance, the vein is entered with a 21-gauge needle.

Once venous access is achieved, two important distances must be measured. The first is the distance from the mid-right atrium to the venotomy site, and the second is the length of the subcutaneous tunnel. Because all catheters come in fixed, predetermined lengths and patients come in all shapes and sizes, the subcutaneous tunnel has to be sized to the patient to ensure the catheter tip lies in the right atrium.

For the first measurement, the tip of the wire is placed in the right atrium under fluoroscopic guidance. The wire is bent as it exits the introducer catheter; this measured distance is used in a later step to determine the length of the subcutaneous tunnel. Next, a 0.035-inch guidewire is advanced until the tip is in the caudal inferior vena cava in order to facilitate advancement of the large and stiff introducer sheath. Sufficient purchase of the wire must be gained by placing it distally in order to prevent the wire from deviating into the mediastinum as the sheath is advanced. The bent wire is used to determine the length of the subcutaneous tunnel by the following method. The tip of the wire and the tip of the catheter are placed end to end. The distance from the right atrium to the venotomy site, as measured to the bend in the wire, is subtracted from the tip of the catheter. As measured on the catheter, the length of the subcutaneous tunnel is the distance remaining on the catheter from the bend in the wire to the Dacron cuff on the catheter. By making this measurement, one can be assured that the catheter cuff will lie just within the subcutaneous tunnel, making eventual catheter removal far easier.

The catheter insertion kits come with one of a variety of tunneling tools, but a hemostat often is used to create the subcutaneous tunnel. The tunneling tool can then be used to thread the catheter through the tunnel once it is created.

Care must be taken while advancing the dilator-sheath system to ensure that the sheath stays within the anatomic boundaries of the central venous system, because the sheaths are long and stiff enough to puncture the mediastinum. Once the catheter is tunneled and the dilator-sheath system is placed into the superior vena cava, the distal portion of the catheter is advanced into the venous system using standard technique. Once the catheter is delivered, the skin incision over the venotomy site is closed with a single subcutaneous, absorbable suture, and the catheter is sutured to the skin at the tunnel exit site. The ports are flushed with heparinized saline (1,000 U/mL), and a sterile dressing is applied before the sterile field is broken.

MANAGEMENT OF COMPLICATIONS

Hemodialysis catheters are subject to a number of delayed complications. Most frequently, complications include thrombosis, fibrin sheath formation and infection. Catheter tip thrombosis and fibrin sheath formation are manifested by the inability to flush or aspirate the catheter as well as decreased flow rates during dialysis. Many dialysis units have established protocols for managing these complications in order to reestablish catheter patency. Protocols include reversing the ports (i.e., using the arterial port to return blood and the venous port to aspirate) and the use of thrombolytic agents. If these maneuvers are not successful, the catheter may need to be replaced. Catheters can be replaced either by removing the existing catheter and placing a new one at a different site, or by exchanging the existing catheter for a new one over a guidewire (17). Guidewire exchange preserves the venotomy site, which may be an important consideration in the hemodialysis population. Hemodialysis patients are subject to repeated placement of catheters during the course of their lifetimes, and each catheter insertion subjects the vein to trauma and the risk of fibrosis and stricture. Minimizing the number of catheter insertions preserves potential sites for access over the patient's lifetime (17,18). As discussed later in this section, preservation of the venotomy site becomes especially important when managing catheter-related bacteremia and infection.

Management of fibrin sheath formation is a somewhat debatable topic. The formation of a fibrin sheath begins immediately after a catheter is placed. Over the course of weeks to months the sheath can reduce flow rates within the catheter or progress to completely occlude the catheter. Various interventions to salvage catheter function exist, including placement of a new catheter at a different site, stripping the sheath with a snare, using a tip deflecting wire inside the catheter to disrupt the sheath, and guidewire exchange of the catheter (17,19,20). Preservation of the venotomy, as stated previously, is an important consideration when choosing a method of treating a malfunctioning catheter. Placement of a new catheter at a different site means a new venotomy, and a potential new stricture or occlusion making a new venotomy the least desirable alternative. Stripping the sheath with a snare was first described in the literature in 1995; controlled studies have shown the method to be safe and effective at restoring patency to failing catheters (19). However, stripping the sheath requires a puncture in the groin and is technically more demanding than other methods. In addition, if the catheter is adjacent to the vessel wall, it may be impossible to slide the snare around the catheter tip. Using a tip-deflecting wire disrupts the sheath, but does not completely remove it (21). Guidewire exchange preserves the venotomy site, is technically simple, and compares favorably with new catheter placement in terms of catheter longevity (17,18).

Pharmacologic intervention includes using thrombolytic agents to disrupt the catheter tip fibrin cap (21). Three methods can be used with thrombolytic agents. The first method consists of a simple "load and lock" procedure, in which the catheter lumens are filled with tissue plasminogen activator (TPA) at a concentration of 1 mg/mL. If ineffective, a prolonged catheter infusion with TPA may be required, infusing low volumes of highly concentrated TPA through both lumens. The protocol used at my institution consists of a 4-hour infusion, 2 hours per lumen, infusing 1 mg of TPA in 10 mL of normal saline per hour. The final method of using TPA is by including the thrombolytic agent in the dialysate during dialysis treatments (22).

Catheter-related bacteremia and infections are perhaps the most vexing complications associated with hemodialysis catheters. Bacterial colonization of the catheter can lead to bacteremia and septic episodes; left untreated, the bacteremia puts the patient at risk for septic emboli, leading to pulmonary abscesses and endocarditis. The likelihood of catheter bacterial colonization increases with the amount of time the catheter is in place (20). Catheter hubs are manipulated during hemodialysis, exposing the inner lumens to skin flora. In a prospective study, Dittmer showed that colonization was universally present by 16 weeks. The risk of subsequent bacteremia was related to time left in place and the degree of bacterial colonization (20). Catheter colonization is also related to fibrin sheaths, which likely form a matrix for bacterial colonization (23). Treating the fibrin cap may be necessary to adequately treat the infection.

The management of catheter-related bacteremia is a controversial subject (24–27). Opinions vary widely whether removing the catheter is required at the first sign of sepsis or whether the patient can be managed without removing the catheter. As noted previously, preserving venous access is a priority when managing hemodialysis catheters because every new venipuncture puts the patient at risk for venous stricture and occlusion. In 1997 the National Kidney Foundation compiled a set of guidelines based on the best available scientific evidence and the consensus opinions of nephrologists and other specialists. The guidelines, termed the Dialysis Outcome Quality Initiative (DOQI), outlined protocols for managing catheter-related bacteremia (28). In summary, for suspected episodes of catheter-related bacteremia, the patient should be started on intravenous antibiotics and the catheter left in place. If the septic episode improves after 48 hours, the patient is continued on antibiotics and the catheter exchanged over a guidewire as soon as the patient becomes afebrile. If there is no improvement, the catheter is removed and a temporary catheter placed at a different site. Resolution of the septic episode must be documented by negative blood cultures obtained on two separate days before a new tunneled catheter is placed. Treating the septic episode with antibiotics and guidewire exchange salvages close to 50% of tunneled lines and is more effective than antibiotics alone (27). The DOQI guidelines emphasize preservation of the venotomy, while exposing the patient to minimal additional risk during a catheter-related septic episode.

REFERENCES

1. Kherlakian GM, Roedersheimer LR, Arbaugh JJ, et al. Comparison of autogenous fistula versus expanded polytetrafluoroethylene graft fistula for angioaccess in hemodialysis. *Am J Surg* 1986;152:238–243.
2. Albers F. Causes of hemodialysis access failure. *Adv Ren Replace Ther* 1994;1:107–118.
3. Zibari GB, Rohr MS, Landreneau MD, et al. Complications from permanent hemodialysis vascular access. *Surgery* 1988;104:681–686.

4. Broviac JW, Cole JJ, Scribner BH. A silicone rubber catheter for prolonged parenteral alimentation; *Surg Gynecol Obstet* 1973;136:602–606.

5. Hickman RO, Buckner CD, Clift RA, et al. A modified right atrial catheter for access to the venous system in marrow transplant recipients. *Surg Gynecol Obstet* 1979;148:871–875.

6. Moss AH, McLaughlin MM, Lempet KD, et al. Use of a silicone catheter with a Dacron cuff for dialysis short-term vascular access. *Am J Kidney Dis* 1988;12: 492–498.

7. Hassell DD, Vesley TM, Pilgram TK, et al. Initial performance of Tesio hemodialysis catheters. *JVIR* 1999; 10:553–558.

8. Leblanc M, Bosc JY, Vaussenat F, et al. Effective blood flow and recirculation rates in internal jugular vein twin catheters: measurement by ultrasound velocity dilution. *Am J Kidney Dis* 1998;31:87–92.

9. Millner MR, Kerns SR, Hawkins IF, et al. Tesio twin catheter system: a new catheter for hemodialysis. *AJR* 1995;164:1519–1520.

10. Trerotola SO, Shah H, Johnson M, et al. Randomized comparison of high-flow versus conventional hemo-dialysis catheters. *JVIR* 1999;10:1032–1038.

11. Mankus RA, Ash S, Sutton JM. Comparison of blood flow rates and hydraulic resistance between the Mahurkar catheter, the Tesio twin catheter, and the Ash split cath. *ASAIO* 1998;99:532–534.

12. Konner K. Subclavian haemodialysis access: is it still justified in 1995? *Nephrol Dial Transplant* 1995;10: 1988–1999.

13. Cimochowski GE, Worley E, Rutherford WE, et al. Superiority of the internal jugular over the subclavian access for temporary dialysis. *Nephron* 1990;54: 154–161.

14. Lameris JS, Post PJM, Zonderland HM, et al. Percutaneous placement of Hickman catheters: comparison of sonographically guided and blind techniques. *AJR* 1990;155:1097–1099.

15. Mallory DL, McGee WT, Shawker TH, et al. Ultrasound guidance improves the success rate of internal jugular vein cannulation. *Chest* 1990;98:157–160.

16. Robertson LJ, Mauro MA, Jaques PF. Radiologic placement of Hickman catheters. *Radiology* 1989;170: 1007–1009.

17. Duszak R, Haskel ZJ, Thomas-Hawkins C, et al. Replacement of failing tunneled hemodialysis catheters through pre-existing subcutaneous tunnels: a comparison of catheter function and infection rates for *de novo* placements and over-the-wire exchanges. *JVIR* 1998; 9:321–327.

18. Garofalo RS, Zaleski GX, Lorenz JM, et al. Exchange of poorly functioning tunneled permanent hemodialysis catheters. *AJR* 1999;173:155–158.

19. Brady PS, Spence LD, Levitin A, et al. Efficacy of percutaneous fibrin sheath stripping in restoring patency of tunneled hemodialysis catheters. *AJR* 1999;173: 1023–1027.

20. Dittmer ID, Sharp D, McNulty CAM, et al. A prospective study of central venous hemodialysis catheter colonization and peripheral bacteremia. *Clin Nephrol* 1999;51:34–39.

21. Knelson MH, Hudson ER, Suhocki PV, et al. Functional restoration of occluded central venous catheters: new interventional techniques. *J Vasc Intervent Radiol* 1995;6:623–627.

22. Twardowski ZJ. High-dose intradialytic urokinase to restore the patency of permanent central vein hemodialysis catheters. *Am J Kidney Dis* 1998;31: 841–847.

23. Raad II, Luna M, Khalil SM, et al. The relationship between the thrombotic and infectious complications of central venous catheters. *JAMA* 1994;271:1014–1016.

24. Beathard GA; Management of bacteremia associated with tunneled-cuffed hemodialysis catheters. *J Am Soc Nephrol* 1999;10:1045–1049.

25. Saad TF, Bacteremia associated with tunneled, cuffed hemodialysis catheters. *Am J Kidney Dis* 1999;34: 1114–1124.

26. Schwab SJ, Beathard G; The hemodialysis catheter conundrum: hate living with them, but can't live without them. *Kidney Int* 1999;56:1–17.

27. Robinson D, Suhocki P, Schwab SJ. Treatment of infected tunneled venous access hemodialysis catheters with guidewire exchange. *Kidney Int* 1998;53:1792–1794.

28. NKF-DOQI Guidelines. *Am J Kidney Dis* 1997;30 (suppl):176–177.

Central Venous Access
Edited by Charles E. Ray, Jr.
Lippincott Williams & Wilkins, Philadelphia © 2001.

9

Peripherally Inserted Central Catheters

Atul K. Gupta, MD

Department of Radiology, Roswell Park Cancer Institute;
State University of New York (SUNY)—Buffalo, Buffalo, New York 14263

The use of long-term central venous catheters (CVCs) continues to increase. Recently, there has been a shift from inpatient to outpatient care, and a concomitant increase in longer term intravenous (IV) therapy. For intermediate and long-term indications, catheters with increased longevity are replacing traditional nontunneled subclavian and internal jugular temporary CVCs. These catheter types include peripherally inserted central catheters (PICCs), tunneled CVCs, and subcutaneous ports.

TERMINOLOGY

By definition, a CVC is one whose tip is located in a central vessel (i.e., the thoracic vena cava). A PICC is a catheter inserted via a peripheral vein whose tip terminates in the vena cava. By contrast, a mid-clavicular catheter is a catheter whose tip resides in the brachiocephalic vein, subclavian vein, or proximal axillary vein. Similarly, if the tip terminates in the proximal portion of the arm, the catheter is termed a midline catheter, and also is not considered a central catheter. Placement of mid-clavicular or midline catheters may be necessary for patients who cannot undergo radiography (e.g., those placed in a home health-care setting), or for patients with known central venous occlusion. In other patients, however, a central catheter should be placed due to the increased incidence of complications noted with mid-clavicular or midline catheters (1,2).

QUALIFICATIONS

The Intravenous Nurse Society (INS) supports the premise that a licensed physician or licensed registered nurse (as determined by state regulations) that is appropriately trained and has demonstrated competency can insert a PICC (3). PICCs placed at the bedside are introduced via a visible or palpable antecubital vein and are blindly advanced, hopefully terminating in the superior vena cava (SVC). A chest radiograph follows the placement procedure to confirm position of the catheter tip in the SVC. If not involved from the start, radiologists are typically consulted when a superficial vein is not visible or palpable in the antecubital region, when the operator is unable to advance the catheter, or when the catheter tip is malpositioned following bedside placement.

VENOUS ANATOMY

The veins of the upper extremity are defined as superficial and deep. The deep system consists of the radial, ulnar, and interosseous veins in the forearm, and the paired brachial veins in the upper arm. The superficial system consists of the cephalic and basilic veins in the forearm and upper arm. The deep vessels are usually smaller than the superficial veins; the majority of the blood flow from the upper extremity is via the superficial veins. The venous anatomy of the upper extremities is discussed in more detail in Chapter 2.

Important anatomic relationships determine which veins are more or less amenable to use during PICC placement. The confluence of the cephalic vein into the axillary vein usually approaches 90 degrees, on occasion making it difficult to manipulate a wire around this venous confluence. The brachial vein represents the main deep vein in the upper arm. It courses in a common fascial sheath with the brachial artery and nerve. The confluence of the radial, ulnar, and interosseous veins of the forearm forms the brachial vein. Due to the deep location of the vein, the proximity of the adjacent artery, the smaller size of the normally paired veins, and the location of the vein within a fascial sheath, the brachial vein is not typically used as the primary vein of choice in PICC placement. Conversely, the nearly straight course and superficial location of the basilic vein makes this vein the preferable access vein for PICC placement.

INDICATIONS

There are a wide variety of indications for PICC placement (Table 9.1). The catheters improve patient comfort by obviating the need for repeated venipunctures for IV therapy or blood draws. They also are convenient for postprocedure care by the patient because the location on the upper arm is easier to clean and maintain than a site on the upper chest or neck, which may be viewed only with the aid of a mirror. The referring physicians and patients appreciate the lower risks of a PICC when compared with subclavian or jugular catheter placements. Pneumothorax, which may be life threatening and may require a tube thoracostomy, does not occur with PICC placements. Additionally, bleeding during catheter placement, which may be significant especially in thrombocytopenic or coagulopathic patients, may be difficult to control in the chest or neck and may necessitate surgical intervention. During placement of a PICC, manual pressure over the bleeding vessel in the arm typically controls bleeding complications.

The duration for which PICCs may be used varies within the literature. In multiple studies,

TABLE 9.1. *PICC indications*

Patient comfort (no need for repeated needle punctures)
Convenience (easy for patient to take care of)
Decreased risk (less chance of pneumothorax or bleeding complications)
Long-term access
Home therapy (safe, reliable, easy to manage)
Miscellaneous (frequent blood sampling, poor peripheral veins for access)

PICC, peripherally inserted central catheter.

PICCs have been shown to have mean dwell times of 17 to 73 days (range 0–432 days) (2–5). This makes them ideal for intermediate or occasionally for long-term therapy. They do not require frequent changes, and because they are safe, reliable, and easy to manage, they are an ideal choice for outpatient therapy. PICCs are typically placed for patients who will require IV therapy for 2 weeks to 2 months. If shorter therapy is required, either peripheral angiocatheters or a temporary CVC may be used; if longer therapy is required, a tunneled or implantable device is typically indicated.

CONTRAINDICATIONS

Peripherally inserted central catheters are not the best venous access option for all patients (Table 9.2). When the patient does not have a continuous arm vein (e.g., due to stricture, thrombosis, surgical ligation, etc.), then a PICC

TABLE 9.2. *PICC contraindications*

Absolute contraindications	Relative contraindications
Peripheral venous obstruction	Septicemia
Inadequate line care arrangements (home care)	Coagulopathy
Need for extensive blood products	Ipsilateral paralysis or mastectomy
	Chronic central venous occlusion
	End-stage renal disease
	Skin burns, infection, or other other dermatologic disorder

PICC, peripherally inserted central catheter.

line may be difficult to place. Also, because a PICC is a foreign body designed for long-term access, it may become colonized in patients with bacteremia; therefore, it may not be be the best choice for venous access in some patients until the infection is resolved (4). If a patient cannot manage the postprocedure care of a PICC (e.g., flushes, dressing, and hub changes) or there are inadequate home health-care arrangements, then a PICC should not be used because of risks of septicemia, bleeding, cellulitis, or air embolus (4). Therefore, it is important to determine who will provide postprocedure care for the PICC prior to its placement. Because PICCs have a small inner diameter and a long length, one of their greatest drawbacks is their limited flow rate, making them unreliable for infusing blood products. The viscosity of packed red blood cells (PRBCs) varies greatly from one unit to the next; therefore, one unit of PRBCs may infuse well while another may not infuse at all. Hence, an alternative means of venous access should be considered if a patient requires extensive blood product transfusions (4,6).

Extensive burns, cellulitis, or a diffuse dermatologic disorder over the access site may necessitate another means of venous access. Ipsilateral paralysis or mastectomy increases the risk of thrombophlebitis, and placement of a CVC is a relative contraindication. Similarly, chronic central venous occlusion is a relative contraindication, although in many cases the tip of the catheter may be placed just peripheral to the occlusion. In patients with end-stage renal disease, use of upper extremity veins is to be avoided whenever possible because damage to these vessels may prevent creation of a dialysis fistula or graft in the future.

Although any procedure on a patient with a coagulopathy is a risk for bleeding complications, because PICCs are placed into a superficial vein in the arm, catheter placements can be performed with relatively low risk despite a moderate coagulopathy. A prothrombin time within 3 seconds of control, a hematocrit of greater than 30%, a platelet count of greater than 50,000/μL, an international normalized ratio (INR) of less than 1.2, and a partial thromboplastin time of less than 40 seconds are preferred (7).

PREPROCEDURE PREPARATION

A medical history and directed physical examination are essential prior to placement of a venous access device. In particular, a history of allergies, previous surgeries, prior venous access, anemias, and medications should be noted. Review of recent laboratory examinations, including a complete blood count, chemistries, and a coagulation profile, is advisable. An electrocardiogram also may prove advantageous. The most important component of the preprocedure assessment is determining the indication for line placement and the planned duration of its use. In this way, the referring physician may be directed to the correct type of venous access device to meet the needs of the patient.

CATHETER TYPE

A wide variety of PICC sizes and designs are available. No single design has been shown to be clearly superior to the others, and patient or operator preference often determines the type of PICC placed (Table 9.3).

There are two basic catheter tip designs: end-hole and valved (Groshong type).

The end-hole catheter is the most common type used for radiologically guided PICC placement because it can be advanced over a guidewire. End-hole catheters can have single or multiple lumens, and if multiple lumens are present they may be staggered or flush with the catheter tip. A staggered-tip, dual-lumen, end-hole catheter has one lumen exiting the catheter proximal to the tip, and a second lumen terminating at the catheter tip itself. The advantage of the staggered tip is that two incompatible substances can be infused simultaneously, one through each lumen. However, if the tip is trimmed during the placement procedure, to ensure proper catheter length the staggered tip is removed.

The Groshong valve tip does not have an end hole, so it cannot be advanced or exchanged over a guidewire without damaging the valve

TABLE 9.3. *Peripherally inserted central catheters and midline catheters*

Manufacturer	Product	Material	Single lumen sizes available (diameter:length)	Multiple lumen sizes available (diameter:length)	Midline available	Exit ports (for multiple lumens)
Arrow International, Inc., www.arrowintl. com	PICC	Poly-urethane	3.0 Fr *(20 ga)*: 55 cm 4.0 Fr *(18 ga)*: 55 cm 5.0 Fr *(16 ga)*: 55 cm 5.0 Fr *(16 ga)*: 70 cm 4.0 Fr *(18 ga)*: 50 cm 5.0 Fr *(16 ga)*: 50 cm	4.0 Fr *(22/22 ga)*: 55 cm 5.0 Fr *(18/20 ga)*: 55 cm 4.0 Fr *(22/22 ga)*: 50 cm 5.0 Fr *(18/20 ga)*: 50 cm	3.0 Fr 4.0 Fr 5.0 Fr	Staggered and trimmable available
Bard Access Systems, Inc., www.bardaccess. com	Groshong®	Silicone	3.0 Fr *(20 ga)*: 60 cm 4.0 Fr *(18 ga)*: 60 cm	5.0 Fr *(19/20 ga)*: 57 cm 5.0 Fr *(19/20 ga)*: 60 cm	3.0 Fr 4.0 Fr	Staggered
	Per-Q-Cath Plus	Silicone	2.0 Fr *(23 ga)*: 30 cm 3.0 Fr *(20 ga)*: 65 cm 4.0 Fr *(18 ga)*: 65 cm 5.0 Fr *(16 ga)*: 65 cm	4.0 Fr *(23/19 ga)*: 65 cm 5.0 Fr *(19/19 ga)*: 65 cm 6.0 Fr *(18/18 ga)*: 65 cm	2.0 Fr 3.0 Fr 4.0 Fr 5.0 Fr *(single lumen)*	Non-staggered
	Poly Per-Q-Cath	Poly-urethane	2.0 Fr *(23 ga)*: 30 cm 3.0 Fr *(20 ga)*: 63 cm 4.0 Fr *(18 ga)*: 63 cm 5.0 Fr *(16 ga)*: 63 cm	4.0 Fr *(21/19 ga)*: 63 cm 5.0 Fr *(18/18 ga)*: 63 cm 6.0 Fr *(17/17 ga)*: 63 cm	2.0 Fr 3.0 Fr 4.0 Fr 5.0 Fr *(single lumen)*	Non-staggered
B. Braun Medical, Inc., www.bbraunusa. com	Accuguide	Poly-urethane	3.0 Fr *(22 ga)*: 60 cm 3.0 Fr *(22 ga)*: 45 cm 4.0 Fr *(18 ga)*: 45 cm 4.0 Fr *(18 ga)*: 60 cm 5.0 Fr *(16 ga)*: 60 cm	4.0 Fr *(18/20 ga)*: 55 cm 5.0 Fr *(17/19 ga)*: 55 cm	3.0 Fr 4.0 Fr *(single lumen)* 4.0 Fr 5.0 Fr *(dual lumen)*	Formed tip and staggered
BD Medical Systems, www.bd.com/ infusion	First PICC	Silicone	1.9 Fr *(24–22 ga)*: 50 cm 2.8 Fr *(20–19 ga)*: 50 cm 3.0 Fr *(20–19 ga)*: 65 cm 4.0 Fr *(19–17 ga)*: 65 cm 5.0 Fr *(18–15 ga)*: 65 cm	5.0 Fr *(15 ga)*: 65 cm	3.0 Fr 4.0 Fr 5.0 Fr *(single and dual lumen)*	Non-staggered
	BD L-Cath	Poly-urethane	1.2 Fr *(28–24 ga)*: 8 cm 1.2 Fr *(28–24 ga)*: 14 cm 1.2 Fr *(28–24 ga)*: 20 cm 1.2 Fr *(28–24 ga)*: 25 cm 1.9 Fr *(24–20 ga)*: 8 cm 1.9 Fr *(24–20 ga)*: 15 cm 1.9 Fr *(24–20 ga)*: 19 cm 1.9 Fr *(24–20 ga)*: 25 cm 1.9 Fr *(24–20 ga)*: 30 cm 2.6 Fr *(20–19 ga)*: 20 cm 2.6 Fr *(20–19 ga)*: 20 cm 3.0 Fr *(20–18 ga)*: 20 cm 3.0 Fr *(20–18 ga)*: 60 cm	2.6 Fr *(22/23–19 ga)*: 60 cm 3.5 Fr *(20/21–17 ga)*: 60 cm 5.0 Fr *(18/19–16 ga)*: 60 cm	2.6 Fr 3.0 Fr 3.5 Fr 5.0 Fr	Non-staggered

TABLE 9.3. *(Continued)*

Manufacturer	Product	Material	Single lumen sizes available (diameter:length)	Multiple lumen sizes available (diameter:length)	Midline available	Exit ports (for multiple lumens)
BD Medical Systems, *(cont.)*	BD L-Cath	Poly-urethane	3.5 Fr *(18–17 ga)*: 20 cm 3.5 Fr *(18–17 ga)*: 60 cm 5.0 Fr *(16–14 ga)*: 20 cm 5.0 Fr *(16–14 ga)*: 60 cm			
	BD L-Cath EX	Poly-urethane	1.9 Fr *(24–20 ga)*: 8 cm 1.9 Fr *(24–20 ga)*: 15 cm 2.6 Fr *(20–19 ga)*: 8 cm 2.6 Fr *(20–19 ga)*: 15 cm 3.5 Fr *(18–17 ga)*: 8 cm 3.5 Fr *(18–17 ga)*: 15 cm	None	Yes	NA
Boston Scientific/ Vascular, www.bsci.com	Vaxcel	Poly-urethane	4.0 Fr *(18 ga)*: 60 cm 5.0 Fr *(16 ga)*: 60 cm	5.0 Fr *(16 ga)*: 60 cm 6.0 Fr *(13 ga)*: 60 cm	None	Non-staggered
Catheter Innovations, Inc., www.pasv.com	PASV PICC	Silicone	3.0 Fr *(20 ga)*: 60 cm 4.0 Fr *(18 ga)*: 60 cm 5.0 Fr *(17 ga)*: 60 cm 6.0 Fr *(16 ga)*: 60 cm	5.0 Fr *(18.5/18.5 ga)*: 60 cm *(dual lumen)* 6.0 Fr *(18/18 ga)*: 60 cm *(dual lumen)*	3.0 Fr *(20 ga)*: 20 cm 4.0 Fr *(18 ga)*: 20 cm 5.0 Fr *(17 ga)*: 20 cm 6.0 Fr *(16 ga)*: 20 cm 5.0 Fr *(18.5/ 18.5 ga)*: 20 cm *(dual lumen)* 6.0 Fr *(18/ 18 ga)*: 20 cm *(dual lumen)*	Non-staggered
Cook Critical Care, www.cookgroup.com	C-PICS	Silicone	3.0 Fr *(20–19 ga)*: 50 cm 4.0 Fr *(18–17 ga)*: 60 cm 5.0 Fr *(16–15 ga)*: 60 cm	6.0 Fr *(20/18–13 ga)*: 50 cm 7.0 Fr *(18/16–11 ga)*: 50 cm	None	Non-staggered
	UPICS	Poly-urethane	4.0 Fr *(18–22 ga)*: 60 cm 5.0 Fr *(16–22 ga)*: 60 cm			
HDC Corporation, www.hdccorp.com	V-Cath	Silicone	2.0 Fr *(23–20 ga)*: 25 cm 2.0 Fr *(23–20 ga)*: 40 cm 3.0 Fr *(20–17 ga)*: 60 cm 3.8 Fr *(18–16 ga)*: 60 cm	3.9 Fr *(20/20 ga)*: 60 cm 5.0 Fr *(18/18–15 ga)*: 50 cm 5.0 Fr *(18/18–15 ga)*: 60 cm 7.0 Fr *(16/16–11 ga)*: 60 cm	2.0 Fr *(23 ga)* 3.0 Fr *(20 ga)* 3.9 Fr *(20/ 20 ga)* *(dual lumen)*	Staggered and non-staggered

TABLE 9.3. *(Continued)*

Manufacturer	Product	Material	Single lumen sizes available (diameter:length)	Multiple lumen sizes available (diameter:length)	Midline available	Exit ports (for multiple lumens)
HDC Corporation, *(cont.)*	V-Cath	Silicone	4.0 Fr *(17–14 ga)*: 60 cm 5.0 Fr *(16–14 ga)*: 60 cm		4.0 Fr *(17 ga)* 5.0 Fr *(18/18 ga)* *(dual lumen)*	
Johnson & Johnson Medical, Inc., www.jn medical. com	BIOVUE® PICC and Midline Catheters with the PROTEC-TIV® Safety Introducer	Poly-urethane	2.0 Fr *(24–21 ga)*: 30 cm 3.0 Fr *(20–19 ga)*: 60 cm 4.0 Fr *(18–17 ga)*: 60 cm	4.0 Fr *(18–17 ga)*: 20 cm 4.0 Fr *(18–17 ga)*: 60 cm 5.0 Fr *(16–15 ga)*: 60 cm	3.0 Fr *(20–19 ga)*: 20 cm 4.0 Fr *(18–17 ga)*: 20 cm *(single lumen)* 4.0 Fr *(18–19 ga)*: 20 cm *(dual lumen)*	Non-staggered
SIMS Deltec, Inc., www.deltec. com	CliniCath	Poly-urethane	2.0 Fr *(24 ga)*: 50 cm 2.0 Fr *(24 ga)*: 30 cm 3.0 Fr *(20 ga)*: 65 cm 4.0 Fr *(18 ga)*: 65 cm 5.0 Fr *(16 ga)*: 65 cm	4.0 Fr *(18 ga)*: 20 cm 4.0 Fr *(18 ga)*: 65 cm 5.0 Fr *(16 ga)*: 65 cm	2.0 Fr *(24 ga)*: 20 cm 3.0 Fr *(20 ga)*: 20 cm 4.0 Fr *(18 ga)*: 20 cm	Non-staggered and trimable
Vygon Corporation, www.vygonusa. com	LifeVac PICC	Silicone	3.0 Fr *(20–17 ga)*: 60 cm 4.0 Fr *(18–16 ga)*: 60 cm 5.0 Fr *(16–14 ga)*: 60 cm	4.0 Fr *(18/20–16 ga)*: 60 cm 4.5 Fr *(18/18–14 ga)*: 60 cm	None	NA
	LifeVac Midline	Flexane	None	None	3.0 Fr *(17 ga)* 4.0 Fr *(17 ga)*	NA
	Premicath	Flexane	1.1 Fr *(27–24 ga)*: 8 cm 1.1 Fr *(27–24 ga)*: 20 cm	None	Yes	NA
	Nutriline	Flexane	2.0 Fr *(23–20 ga)*: 30 cm	None	None	NA
	E.C.C.	Silicone	2.0 Fr *(23–19 ga)*: 30 cm	None	Yes	NA

PICC, peripherally inserted central catheter; NA, not available.
Reprinted from *Infusion* 2000:44,46,48,50; with permission.

mechanism. This catheter design has a slit near the tip, which functions as a valve to prevent spontaneous backflow of blood into the catheter lumen. Because there is no blood within the catheter, a heparin flush is not required, and Groshong type catheters are usually flushed weekly with sterile saline. This benefit provides an excellent alternative for patients with a heparin allergy, heparin-induced thrombocytopenia, or other contraindications to low-dose heparin use.

Although Groshong tip catheters typically prevent blood backflow into the catheter lumen, multiple scenarios may cause valve dysfunction. The valve mechanism may be overcome by an increase in intrathoracic pressure, as with a cough or retching. If a fibrin sheath surrounds the catheter tip, valvular incompetence may occur with aspiration of parts of the fibrin sheath into the valve mechanism itself. Once blood is inside the lumen, clotting may occur because these catheters are not routinely flushed with heparin. The impact of these clots on catheter function is not certain, although intraluminal blood might increase the risk of catheter-related infection because it would provide a rich culture medium in a space isolated from the patient's immune system (7).

Larger lumens improve flow characteristics and by doing so, in theory, should decrease the number of catheter occlusions. Larger lumens, and a greater number of lumens, increase the outer diameter of the catheter, making PICC placement more difficult and more likely to occlude small arm veins. In addition, increasing the number of lumens has been shown to be an independent variable that increases the risk of catheter-related infection (8–10). In an attempt to compromise between intraluminal catheter occlusions and venous occlusions, pediatric patients typically receive a 2 to 4 French (Fr) catheter, whereas adults receive either a 4 to 5 Fr single-lumen catheter or a 5 to 6 Fr dual-lumen PICC. If single-agent therapy is planned (e.g., total parenteral nutrition, single antibiotic agent), then a single-lumen catheter is preferred. Multilumen catheters are reserved for use when multiple simultaneous infusions are needed.

Almost all currently available PICCs are made from silicone or polyurethane compounds. Polyurethane has greater tensile strength than silicone, so a thinner walled catheter can be designed without compromising the inner lumen diameter (Fig. 9.1). Therefore, for the same outer diameter, a larger lumen with better flow characteristics is obtained by using polyurethane instead of silicone (4–6,11,12). However, polyurethane is a stiffer material and theoretically is more likely to cause vascular injury; many polyurethane catheters become softer after placement into the bloodstream, which should decrease the risk of long-term vascular injury (5,11,13). Some formulations of polyure-

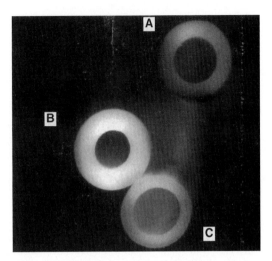

FIG. 9.1. Section of three different 4 French single-lumen peripherally inserted central catheters. Polyurethane **(A)**, silicone **(B)**, and thin-walled polyurethane catheters **(C)**. Note that the lumen of the two polyurethane catheters are larger than for the silicone catheter of the same outer diameter.

thane have been known to become brittle on long-term exposure to blood (4). Despite these concerns, many patients have been able to tolerate polyurethane PICCs for over a year without complications (4,5). Silicone is biocompatible, flexible, and nonthrombogenic, and is associated with a low infection rate (5,14). However, because silicone is not as firm as polyurethane, a smaller inner diameter and lower flow rates are achieved for the same outer diameter. Due to its flexibility and biocompatibility, silicone-based catheters may be more advantageous than polyurethane catheters if the PICC is placed below the elbow joint. By using the softer silicone catheters, the likelihood of catheter fracture from repeated trauma due to elbow flexion should be decreased.

PLACEMENT TECHNIQUES

Although a full surgical scrub for the operator and patient is unnecessary, PICCs should be placed using standard sterile angiographic technique. Placing the catheter in the forearm or antecubital fossa requires a catheter that is unnecessarily long and at increased risk for kinking by flexion of the elbow. The upper arm, therefore, is the preferred location.

Venous access can be obtained by any of four guidance methods: direct visualization/palpation; IV iodinated contrast; IV alternative contrast agents; or ultrasonographic guidance. A small number of patients have a visible or palpable cephalic or basilic vein. In these patients, placement of a tourniquet high on the upper arm allows direct puncture with an angiocath or a micropuncture needle. Subsequently, a 0.018-inch guidewire can be advanced to the right atrium, and using standard catheter and guidewire exchanges, the PICC can be placed without any imaging guidance. It is by this method that PICCs are placed at the bedside by IV nursing teams.

Unfortunately, many patients have no visible or palpable superficial veins. In such cases an upper extremity vein can be opacified by injecting dilute contrast agent into a more peripherally placed IV angiocatheter. This method requires some sort of peripheral IV access, which can usually be accomplished with a small-gauge IV needle in the forearm. Excellent opacification can be obtained with less than 10 mL of contrast agent, after which the vein can be punctured with real-time digital roadmap guidance. In patients with a contrast allergy or renal insufficiency, 10 to 20 mL of carbon dioxide administered via the peripheral IV line can be used to visualize the cephalic or basilic vein (4). A tourniquet high on the upper arm should be used to slow the passage of the gas. The image contrast with carbon dioxide may be poor, so several attempts may be necessary to obtain access to the vein.

In the setting of both a contraindication to iodinated contrast and unavailability of carbon dioxide, gadolinium (gadopentate dimeglumine) may be used as an intravascular contrast agent (4).

The vein also can be punctured with ultrasonographic guidance. A 5- to 7.5-MHz linear array transducer usually provides adequate vascular visualization for obtaining access. Ultrasonography can be a valuable tool in patients with contrast allergy or renal insufficiency.

Many patients have had multiple angiocatheters, and their superficial veins are sclerosed; ultrasonographic evaluation is a useful tool in the initial assessment of the patency of upper arm veins. In the setting of superficial vein occlusion, the brachial vein must be used for PICC placement. Because the brachial artery and vein course together in the same sheath, care must be taken to avoid inadvertent arterial puncture. Although venographic guidance allows good visualization of the venous structures, the adjacent artery is not visualized. Ultrasonography is useful in demonstrating the location of the artery, as well as the vein, theoretically decreasing the risk of an arterial puncture or formation of an arteriovenous fistula. As noted above, at my institution upper arm venous access is first attempted via the basilic vein, then via the cephalic vein, and finally via the brachial vein. This algorithm must, of course, be tailored on a patient-by-patient basis.

In order to decrease the risk of bleeding or damage to adjacent structures, a microaccess system (Cook, Inc., Bloomington, IN, U.S.A.) is used for initial vascular access. Once the vein has been accessed, a guidewire is advanced to the right atrium, which is used to measure the appropriate length for the PICC. Because nearly all PICCs have blunt tips, a peel-away sheath is placed into the accessed vein, after which the catheter is placed in standard fashion. The ideal location for the catheter tip is in the proximal right atrium. During placement, the operator must keep in mind that retraction of the catheter tip may occur, although it is less likely to occur with PICCs than with catheters placed directly via a central vein.

COMPLICATIONS

Every procedure has associated risks and complications, and PICC placements are no exception. PICC-related complications can be categorized as early (procedure related) and delayed (Table 9.4). The overall complication rate for PICCs is approximately 2% to 5% (13, 15,17,19).

Some patients have an allergy to iodinated contrast agents, which may or may not be rec-

TABLE 9.4. *PICC-related complications*

Early complications	Delayed complications
Contrast allergy	Infection
Arterial puncture	Catheter occlusion
Venospasm	Venous thrombosis
Bleeding	Fibrin sheath
Technical failure	Catheter malposition
	Mechanical
	Kinking
	Leak
	Fracture

PICC, peripherally inserted central catheter.
Data from Yagmai B, Owens CA, Warner D. Peripherally inserted central catheters. *Semin Intervent Radiol* 1998;15:305–314; Crowley JJ, Pereira JK, Harris LS, et al. PICCs: experience in 523 children. *Radiology* 1997;204:617–621; Ng PK, Ault MJ, Ellrodt AG, Maldonado L. PICCs in general medicine. *Mayo Clin Proc* 1997;72:225–233; Cardella JF, Cardella K, Bacci N, et al. Cumulative experience with 1273 PICCs at a single institution. *J Vasc Intervent Radiol* 1996;7:5–13; Cardella JF, Lukens ML, Fox PS. Fibrin sheath entrapment of PICCs. *J Vasc Intervent Radiol* 1994;5: 439–442; Bottino J, McCredie KB, Groschel DH, et al. Long-term intravenous therapy with peripherally inserted silicone elasomer central venous catheters in patients with malignant disease. *Cancer* 1979;43: 1937–1943; with permission.

ognized prior to PICC placement. An allergic reaction can be prevented by pretreatment with steroids and benadryl, but avoiding the use of iodinated contrast material altogether by using carbon dioxide, gadolinium, or ultrasonography to visualize the vein may prove to be the easiest option. Because venographic guidance fails to show the brachial artery, occasionally the artery is punctured inadvertently. If immediately recognized, the needle can be removed and bleeding can usually be controlled with direct manual pressure over the arterial puncture site. In patients with an underlying coagulopathy, however, control of the bleeding may prove to be more difficult. In these patients ultrasonographic imaging identify the brachial artery so it can be avoided. Likewise, if the arterial puncture is unrecognized and the arteriotomy is dilated to accept the peel-away sheath, significant hemorrhage may occur.

Spasm of the vein can be a cause of failure to access the vein or prevent advancement of the wire. If the first attempt at venipuncture is un-

successful, or if excessive guidewire manipulation is performed, the vein can undergo severe spasm. One protocol for treating venospasm includes administration of 100 μg of nitroglycerin through the peripheral angiocatheter while simultaneously compressing the venous outflow. This maneuver can be repeated every 5 minutes as long as the patient does not demonstrate any significant systemic side effects of the vasodilator (e.g., systemic hypotension). For prolonged venospasm, administration of heparin should be considered to decrease the risk of superimposed venous thrombosis. Systemic pain medications also may be necessary for severe spasm.

Infectious complications represent one of the most severe forms of delayed PICC complications. Infections may occur secondary to seeding of the PICC or PICC tract during the initial catheter placement due to breakdown in sterile technique. Infections also may occur due to inadequate postprocedure catheter care, such as inappropriate catheter flushes or poor wound site care. Infections vary from mild local infections, such as local erythema and tenderness over the skin site, to life-threatening sepsis. Treatment options vary just as widely from treatment with oral antibiotics to treatment with IV antibiotics and catheter removal.

A catheter occupying nearly the diameter of a peripheral vein causes venous stasis, acting as a nidus for thrombosis of the vein. Using a catheter with the smallest possible outer diameter helps minimize this risk (4). Due to transection of lymphatic channels, patients who have undergone an axillary dissection or mastectomy are at increased risk for lymphedema if the ipsilateral arm is used. If possible, the PICC should be placed on the opposite side of the previous surgery in these patients.

SUMMARY

Many options are available for central venous access. PICCs may be a catheter of choice providing intermediate- to long-term venous access that can be safely and conveniently managed at home. They are associated with increased patient comfort and decreased risks, and can be inexpensively placed at the bedside, by a nurse or physician, or by a radiologist employing various imaging techniques if "blind" placement techniques fail.

REFERENCES

1. Position paper. Midline and midclavicular catheters. *J Intraven Nurs* 1997;20:175–178.
2. Position paper. Peripherally inserted central catheters. *J Intraven Nurs* 1997;20:172–174.
3. Lawson T. Infusion of IV medications and fluids via PICC and midline catheters. *JVAD* 1998;Summer:11–17.
4. Angle JF, Hagspiel KD, Spinose DJ, Matsumoto AH. Peripherally inserted central catheters. *Appl Radiol* 1998;27:31–39.
5. Renner C. Polyurethane vs silicone PICC catheters. *JVAD* 1998;Spring:16–21.
6. Angle JF, Matsumoto AH, Skalok TC, et al. Flow characteristics of peripherally inserted central catheters. *JVIR* 1997;8:569–577.
7. Mayo DJ, Helsabeck CB, Horne MK. Intraluminal clots in Groshong catheters. *JVAD* 1995;1:20–22.
8. Keung YK, Watkins K, Chen SC, et al. Comparative study of infectious complications of different types of chronic central venous access devices. *Cancer* 1994; 73:2832–2837.
9. Early TF, Gregory RT, Wheeler JR, et al. Increased infection rate in double-lumen versus single-lumen Hickman catheters in cancer patients. *South Med J* 1990; 83:34–36.
10. Toltzis P, Goldmann DA. Current issues in central venous catheter infection. *Annu Rev Med* 1990;41: 169–176.
11. Hadaway LC. Comparison of vascular access devices. *Semin Oncol Nurs* 1995;3:154–166.
12. Curelaru I, Gustavsson B, Hansson AH, et al. Material thrombogenicity in central venous catheterization: II. A comparison between plain silicone elastomer, and plain polyethelene, long antebrachial catheters. *Acta Anaesthesiol Scand* 1983;27:158–164.
13. Yagmai B, Owens CA, Warner D. Peripherally inserted central catheters. *Semin Intervent Radiol* 1998;15: 305–314.
14. Braun MA. Image-guided peripheral venous access catheters and implantable ports. *Semin Intervent Radiol* 1994;11:358–365.
15. Crowley JJ, Pereira JK, Harris LS, et al. PICCs: experience in 523 children. *Radiology* 1997;204:617–621.
16. Ng PK, Ault MJ, Ellrodt AG, Maldonado L. PICCs in general medicine. *Mayo Clin Proc* 1997;72:225–233.
17. Cardella JF, Cardella K, Bacci N, et al. Cumulative experience with 1273 PICCs at a single institution. *J Vasc Intervent Radiol* 1996;7:5–13.
18. Cardella JF, Lukens ML, Fox PS. Fibrin sheath entrapment of PICCs. *J Vasc Intervent Radiol* 1994;5:439–442.
19. Bottino J, McCredie KB, Groschel DH, et al. Long-term intravenous therapy with peripherally inserted silicone elastomer central venous catheters in patients with malignant disease. *Cancer* 1979;43:1937–1943.

Central Venous Access
Edited by Charles E. Ray, Jr.
Lippincott Williams & Wilkins, Philadelphia © 2001.

10

Postprocedure Care of Venous Access Devices

Charles E. Ray, Jr., MD and *Pamela D. Paplham, NP

Denver Health Medical Center;
University of Colorado Health Sciences Center, Denver, Colorado 80204
*Roswell Park Cancer Institute, Buffalo, New York 14263

With the increasing incidence of central venous access devices (VADs) being placed by radiologists comes the added responsibility of caring for the devices (and patients with the devices) during the postprocedure period. As opposed to many procedures performed in the radiology department, the radiologist placing VADs must function in many ways as the primary caregiver for patients with regard to their VADs. This added responsibility includes making suggestions to the referring clinical service with which type of device to place, to performing or directing the preprocedure evaluation of potential patients, to placement of the device, and to education and performance of postprocedure care.

Becoming intrinsically involved in the postprocedure care of VADs provides many benefits. First, it provides continuity of care to the patient; if questions arise with regard to the VAD, the patient and referring physician have one individual or team that they know to contact. Second, being involved in the postprocedure care of VADs demonstrates to the referring service that the individual placing the device indeed wishes to become acutely involved in all aspects of VAD care. Third, it allows the radiologist to become more involved with the daily decision-making process with regard to the VAD; in essence, it gets the radiologist "out there" in the clinical world. Finally, by being involved with postprocedure care from the outset, potentially serious complications may be recognized early and corrected before they become severe.

Appropriate postprocedure care is vital to the management of patients with indwelling VADs. It has been shown that postprocedure care delivered by a dedicated skilled nursing team significantly decreases the risk of postprocedure complications (Faubian 29 in Paplham)(1). Postprocedure complications may require early removal of VADs. Complications that may arise in the postprocedure period include but are not limited to infections, catheter occlusions, and venous thromboses. Any of these complications may be severely detrimental to the overall care of the patient. In the severely debilitated patient, such complications may even be life threatening. Other potential outcomes from VAD-related complications include hospitalization of the patient to address the complication; the additional cost, inconvenience, and risk of additional drug therapy (e.g., antibiotics) required to treat the complication; delay in therapy for the underlying disease while the complication is being treated; and the unquantifiable cost to the patient due to the stress of unforeseen therapy required to treat the complication. Although not able to completely avoid complications, appropriate postprocedure care for VADs often decreases the severity of the complication, or in some cases may preclude the complication completely.

Many of the complications noted in the post-procedure period are closely related. For example, it has been shown that a fibrin sheath occurring at the catheter tip predisposes the patient to both venous thrombosis and catheter-related infection (2). Postprocedure complications may require early removal of VAD. By recognizing the complication early and initiating appropriate therapy, the complication can be limited to catheter tip occlusion before it progresses to one of the other more severe complications. In the most extreme example, early recognition and treatment of the complication may save the patient from undergoing catheter removal and subsequent catheter replacement, as well as safeguarding them against the adverse outcomes listed above.

ROUTINE POSTPROCEDURE CARE OF VAD

Immediate Postprocedure Care

In the immediate postprocedure period, the patient should be made aware of certain events that are normal, such as postprocedure pain, or others that may represent early signs of complications, such as worsening postprocedure erythema.

Of particular importance for the patient is the understanding that once the effects of the intraprocedural medications (e.g., lidocaine, narcotics) wear off, the area over the VAD placement may become sore or painful. It is important to inform the patient of the possibility that this may occur within a few hours of the procedure itself, and it is important to explain to the patient the difference between normal postprocedural pain and the pain experienced due to early infection. At my institution, the patient is told prior to the VAD placement that the area around the skin exit site, or the incision site in the case of implantable ports, will become "sore like a bruise" within 12 hours following the procedure. The patient is counseled that the postprocedure pain is normal and normally subsides within 48 hours following VAD placement. Prescriptions for pain medication are not routinely given, but the patient is instructed to take 400 mg of ibuprofen every 4 to

TABLE 10.1. *Clinical signs of abnormal postprocedure pain*

Pain that does not subside within 48 hours
Pain that initially improves, then worsens
Pain not controlled with over-the-counter analgesics
Pain associated with discharge or erythema

6 hours as needed for pain control. If, however, any of the following occur, the patient is instructed to return to the radiology department for clinical assessment: if the pain worsens after it initially improves; if the pain does not completely subside within 48 hours; if the pain is not controlled with ibuprofen; or if the pain is associated with discharge or significant erythema (Table 10.1).

During the initial postprocedure period, patients are instructed to keep the skin insertion site or incision clean and dry. For any external catheter, this practice remains for the entire time the patient has the device in place. For implantable systems (i.e., ports), this procedure is followed until any external sutures are removed, or for 7 to 10 days following implantation if subcuticular sutures or skin adhesives are used.

Long-Term Postprocedure Care

Appropriate postprocedure care involves using correct techniques in everything from changing external hubs to properly accessing devices for blood draws or intravenous infusions. Guidelines for routine postprocedure care for implanted ports and external hub catheters are given in Tables 10.2 and 10.3, respectively.

Routine postprocedure care of VADS revolves around maintenance of certain elements of the device itself. In general terms, routine care can be separated into care of the external catheter hubs; care of needle entry sites for implantable devices; care of the incision or catheter exit site, including dressing changes; and catheter flushes (Fig. 10.1).

Care of External Catheter Hubs

Hubs that are attached to the end of any external catheter, whether the catheter is tunneled

TABLE 10.2.   *Postprocedure care of implanted ports*

Site preparation/needle insertion
1. Explain procedure to patient and warn of needle prick sensation.
2. Wash hands thoroughly.
3. Put on sterile gloves.
4. Paint area with alcohol wipe starting at the port and working outward in a spiral motion over an area 4 to 5 inches in diameter.
5. Repeat step 4 with antiseptic swabs three times.
6. Using a sterile, gloved hand, locate port septum by palpation. Locate the base of the port with nondominant hand. Triangulate port between thumb and first two fingers of nondominant hand. Aim for center point of these three fingers.
7. Insert needle perpendicular to port septum. Advance needle through the skin and septum until reaching the bottom of the reservoir.
8. Verify correct needle placement by blood aspiration.
9. Always flush the port after injection.
10. Perform heparin lock procedure according to guidelines or institutional policy. To reduce potential for blood backflow into the catheter tip and possible clotting, always remove the noncoring needle slowly while injecting the last 0.5 mL of solution. Stabilize the port with two fingers during needle withdrawal.

Heparin or saline lock procedure for implanted ports
1. Explain procedure to the patient and prepare injection site.
2. Attach a 10-mL syringe filled with sterile heparinized (100 U/mL) saline to needle.
3. Aseptically locate and access port.
4. Flush the system. To reduce the potential for blood backflow into the catheter tip and possible catheter clotting, always remove a noncoring needle slowly. Maintain positive pressure in the system by withdrawing the syringe and needle while injecting the last 0.5 mL. Stabilize the port with two fingers during needle withdrawal.
5. For ports with Groshong catheters, use the same procedure, only replace heparinized saline with normal saline.

Recommended flushing volumes for implanted ports
1. For ports not in use: 5 mL heparinized saline, or 5 mL normal saline for Groshong-type catheters.
2. After each infusion of medicine or TPN: 10 mL heparinized saline or 10 mL normal saline for Groshong-type catheters.
3. After blood withdrawal: 20 mL heparinized saline, or 20 mL normal saline for Groshong-type catheters.
Note: Other concentrations of heparinized saline have been found to be effective. Determination of proper concentration and volume should be based on the patient's medical condition, laboratory tests, prior experience, and institutional policy.

Bolus injection through an implanted port
1. Explain the procedure to the patient and prepare injection site.
2. Attach noncoring needle to extension set and 10 mL syringe filled with sterile normal saline. Expel all air and clamp extension.
3. Aseptically locate and access the port.
4. Flush port with 10 mL sterile normal saline. Clamp the extension set and remove the syringe.
5. Connect syringe containing the drug to extension set. Release the clamp and administer injection.
6. Examine the injection site for signs of extravasation. If noted immediately, discontinue the injection and initiate appropriate intervention.
7. When the injection is completed, clamp the extension set.
8. Flush after each injection with 10 mL of sterile normal saline to help prevent interaction between incompatible drugs.
9. Perform heparin lock procedure.
Warning: Do not leave the needle hub open to air while it is in the port or manipulate the needle once it is in the septum.

or not, require routine maintenance, which includes periodic hub changes. The particular hub used varies from institution to institution, but the general rules for maintenance remain the same. Procedures used at my institution for catheter hub care during catheter access for either infusion therapy or blood draws are outlined in Table 10.3. Catheter hubs should be changed every 7 days in order to decrease the likelihood of catheter-related infection; if the hubs are accessed more than three times daily, earlier hub changes should be considered. Pro-

TABLE 10.2. *Continued*

Continuous infusion through an implanted port
1. Explain procedure to the patient and prepare the injection site.
2. Attach noncoring needle to the extension set and 10-mL syringe filled with sterile normal saline. Expel all air and clamp the extension set.
3. Aseptically locate and access the port.
4. Apply antibacterial ointment to injection site and place a rolled gauze pad under the needle hub. Secure the needle with a transparent dressing to help prevent inadvertent dislodgment.
5. Open the clamp and flush the port with sterile normal saline. Clamp the extension set and remove the syringe.
6. Connect fluid delivery system to provide additional security during infusion. Tape all tubing connections.
7. Release clamp and initiate infusion. Examine the infusion site for signs of extravasation. If noted, or the patient experiences pain, immediately discontinue the infusion and initiate appropriate intervention.
8. When the infusion is completed, clamp the extension set and then remove the fluid delivery system.
9. Flush after each infusion with 10 mL sterile normal saline to help prevent interaction between incompatible drugs.
10. Perform heparin lock procedure according to guidelines or institutional policy.
Note: It is recommended that the dressing and infusion components be changed every 24 to 48 hours during infusion therapy.
Blood sampling from an implanted port
1. Explain the procedure to the patient and prepare injection site.
2. Aseptically locate and access port.
3. Flush port with sterile normal saline in 10-mL syringe.
4. Withdraw at least 5 mL of blood and discard syringe.
5. Aspirate desired blood volume into 20-mL syringe.
6. Once sample is obtained, immediately flush system with 20 mL of sterile normal saline.
7. Transfer sample into appropriate blood sample tubes.
8. Perform heparin lock procedure.
Clearing blocked implanted port
1. Explain procedure to patient and prepare injection site.
2. Aseptically locate and access the desired septum with needle attached to 10-mL syringe, void of air and filled with 1.8 mL of 5,000 IU/mL urokinase.
3. Gently instill urokinase solution. Use a gentle push-pull action on the syringe plunger to maximize solution mixing within port and catheter. If strong resistance is felt, do not force entire 1.8 mL into catheter.
4. Leave solution in place for 15 minutes.
5. Attempt to aspirate urokinase and the clot.
6. If the clot cannot be aspirated, repeat the procedure.
7. Once the blockage has been cleared, flush the catheter with at least 20 mL of sterile normal saline.
8. Perform heparin lock procedure.
Dressing change of the implanted port
1. Change dressing with permeable dressing every other day until the incision from placement has healed.
2. Once the incision has healed, no dressing is required.

There are varying types of ports within the implanted port category. Please consult the literature accompanying the port to be sure guidelines for care, use, and maintenance do not vary.
Adapted from Paplham P. Post-procedural care of central venous catheters. *Semin Intervent Radiol* 1998; 297–303.

tocols used in catheter hub changes are also presented in Table 10.3.

Accessing Implantable Devices

Care must be taken in accessing ports to preclude the possibility of introducing an infection during port access or in damaging the port device itself. Regardless of the type of device being accessed, certain rules should be strictly followed.

Strict sterile technique, including wearing sterile gloves and mask, appropriate skin cleansing with a bactericidal solution, and using only sterile needles is mandatory any time the skin is punctured over a port. In addition, only noncoring needles (e.g., Huber needles) of the appropriate length should be used. As opposed to standard needles, noncoring needles have a protected needle hole that guards against the needle damaging the silicone septum over the port

TABLE 10.3. *Postprocedural care of tunneled (permanent) and nontunneled (temporary) catheters*

Catheter irrigation procedure

Routine irrigation is required to maintain catheter patency. Flushing frequencies from twice daily (open-ended catheters) to once weekly (Groshong-type catheters) have been found to be effective. However, flushing after transcatheter administration of TPN, IV fluids, or after medications is recommended to maintain patency.

1. Clean injection cap with alcohol, povidone-iodine wipe, or both.
2. Insert needle of 10-mL syringe containing 5 mL normal saline or 2.5 mL heparinized saline (10 U/mL) into injection cap. Always use a 10-mL or larger syringe and flush slowly to avoid rupturing the catheter.
3. Release clamp.
4. Inject irrigation solution, withdrawing needle from injection cap as last 0.5 mL of solution is infused. Injecting under positive pressure helps to prevent a vacuum, which can pull a small amount of blood into the catheter tip.
5. Close catheter clamp if indicated by hospital procedure.
6. For Broviac catheters: Follow the above procedure except use 2 mL normal saline or 1.5 mL heparinized saline.
7. For Groshong catheters: Follow the above procedure except use 10 mL of normal saline.

Blood withdrawal/aspiration procedure: hub-to-hub technique (syringe)

1. Wash hands thoroughly.
2. Draw 10 mL of normal saline into one 10-mL syringe and 2.5 mL heparinized saline into another 10-mL syringe and set aside.
3. Apply smooth-edged atraumatic clamp to silicone clamping sleeve.
4. Stop any IV fluids infusing through the catheter, including another lumen of the catheter. Remove injection cap/IV tubing from catheter hub.
5. Clean catheter hub with alcohol, povidone-iodine wipe, or both.
6. Attach an empty 10-mL syringe to the catheter hub.
7. Open clamp.
8. Aspirate 5 mL of blood.
9. Reclamp the catheter.
10. Disconnect syringe and discard.
11. Attach an empty 10-mL syringe, open the clamp, and aspirate the sample.
12. Reclamp the catheter.
13. Disconnect the syringe and attach a saline-filled syringe.
14. Open the clamp.
15. Flush the catheter with 10 mL normal saline.
16. Reclamp the catheter.
17. Attach the heparin-filled syringe.
18. Open the clamp.
19. Flush the catheter with 2.5 mL heparinized saline.
20. Reclamp the catheter.
21. Disconnect syringe and clean catheter hub with alcohol, povidone-iodine wipes, or both.
22. Attach new injection cap per injection cap change procedure or attach sterile IV tubing to hub of catheter.
23. Attach 1-inch needle to blood sample syringe to transfer to blood collection tubes.

Note: For Groshong-type catheters, it may be necessary to pause 2 seconds during step 8 to allow the distal valve to open.

Injection cap change

The injection cap should be changed every 7 days, after 18 needle insertions, or per hospital policy to minimize the potential for infection from overuse and leakage of the injection cap.

1. Wash hands.
2. Using aseptic technique, open sterile injection cap package and prefill injection cap with heparinized or normal saline.
3. Hold the hub of the catheter below the level of the patient's heart (prevents manometer effect).
4. Apply smooth-edged atraumatic clamp to silicone clamping sleeve and remove the old injection cap.
5. Clean the outside of the catheter hub with an alcohol wipe, povidone-iodine wipe, or both.
6. Remove the tip protector from the new injection cap and twist the cap clockwise onto the catheter hub.
7. Irrigate the catheter with 2.5 mL heparinized saline, or 5 mL normal saline, following the catheter irrigation procedure (per hospital policy).
8. Tape the connection (per hospital policy).

TABLE 10.3. *Continued*

Dressing change procedure

Dressing changes are required to prevent infection of the central venous catheter. Gauze and tape dressings are recommended every Monday, Wednesday, and Friday, or when the dressing becomes soiled, damp, or loosened. Transparent dressings are recommended every 7 days and as needed if loosened.

Note: If the granulocyte count is less than 200/mm, daily dressing changes should be considered. Gauze and tape dressings are recommended for the first 1 or 2 weeks after placement until the cuff is healed because of exudate from the exit site during the healing process.

1. Wash hands.
2. Carefully remove the old dressing and discard. Avoid tugging on the catheter, or the use of scissors, or other sharp objects near the catheter.
3. Inspect the catheter exit site for swelling, redness, or exudate.
4. Wash hands.
5. Put on sterile gloves.
6. Clean the catheter exit site with an alcohol swabstick, starting at the exit site and spiraling outward until a circle at least 3 inches in diameter has been covered. Do not return to the catheter exit site with the same swabstick/applicator. Repeat with the remaining two swabsticks.
7. Repeat step 6 with three povidone-iodine swabsticks.
8. Allow povidone-iodine to dry at least 2 minutes.
9. Gently clean the outside of the catheter with the inside surface of an alcohol wipe, starting from the exit site to the catheter hub. Prevent pulling on the catheter by holding the catheter at the exit site with one alcohol wipe and cleaning with another alcohol wipe.
10. Pat the exit site with sterile gauze to remove any excess povidone-iodine. Apply a small amount of povidone-iodine ointment to the catheter exit site (optional).
11. Apply a split 2 × 2 inch gauze over the catheter exit site for gauze and tape dressings. For transparent dressings, apply transparent dressing by centering it over the catheter exit site (go to step 15 for transparent dressings).
12. Top with a 2 × 2 inch gauze.
13. If a protective dressing wipe or swabstick is used, apply it to the skin to be taped around the periphery of the gauze and allow to dry completely.
14. Cover gauze and 1 inch of surrounding skin with tape or apply transparent dressing by centering it over the catheter exit site.
15. Loop catheter tubing and tape it securely to the dressing or skin (prevents pulling on the catheter).

Troubleshooting of Hickman, Broviac, and Leonard catheters

Clearing occluded catheters

1. Wash hands.
2. Apply smooth-edged atraumatic clamp to silicone clamping sleeve.
3. Remove injection cap, attach an empty 10-mL cc syringe, release clamp, and attempt to aspirate. If aspirate is successful, withdraw clots, clamp catheter, and attach saline-filled syringes. Release clamp and flush catheter with 10 mL normal saline.
4. Clamp catheter and replace cap per Injection Cap Change Procedure.
5. If aspiration is unsuccessful, draw up enough urokinase (5,000 IU/mL) into a 10-mL syringe to equal the internal volume of the catheter.
6. Aseptically attach the urokinase-filled syringe to the catheter hub. Release the clamp and slowly and gently inject the urokinase solution into the catheter. To avoid catheter rupture, do not force entire amount into the catheter.
7. Leave 10-mL syringe attached to the catheter. Do not attempt to aspirate for 30 to 60 minutes.
8. After 30 to 60 minutes, attempt to aspirate the urokinase and residual clot. If unsuccessful, repeat the urokinase instillation.
9. When patency is restored, aspirate 5 cc of blood to assure removal of all drug and clots.
10. Clamp catheter, remove blood-filled syringe, and replace it with a 10-mL syringe.
11. Clamp catheter and remove syringe.
12. Attach sterile heparin-filled injection cap and flush catheter with heparin or saline per Catheter Irrigation Procedure.

reservoir (Fig. 10.1). Using the appropriate needle length keeps the needle from moving to and fro while inside the port septum, decreasing the likelihood of damage to the septum by the needle causing a rent or tear in the septum itself.

There is currently a commercially available implantable device which is significantly differ-

ent from the other currently available devices. The Cathlink system (Bard Access Systems, Salt Lake City, UT, U.S.A.) allows puncture of an implantable port by using standard intravenous cannulas instead of noncoring needles. A series of septa and bends in the port-catheter system prevent damage to the port system when

TABLE 10.3. *Continued*

Aspiration difficulties/catheter occlusion

1. Visually check catheter for any exterior kinks, or constricting sutures. Check operative report, or with placement physician for placement of sutures.
2. If no resistance to infusion is felt, attempt to flush with 10 mL normal saline. Then pull back gently on the syringe plunger 2 to 3 mL, pause and proceed with aspiration.
3. If resistance to infusion is felt, check for signs of extravasation. If present, notify physician of possible catheter leakage or transection. If not present, proceed to step 4.
4. Attempt to aspirate with a 20-mL syringe (creates a greater vacuum).
5. Move the patients arm, shoulder, and head to see if a change in position will allow aspiration. If aspiration can only be accomplished with the patient in a certain position, the patient should be examined to see if the catheter has been placed in the "pinch-off" area.
6. Instill urokinase per clearing occluded catheters procedure.
7. If blood still cannot be aspirated, a chest x-ray, contrast study, or both, may be necessary to confirm catheter position. If the catheter tip is not in the superior vena cava, it should be repositioned or replaced.
8. If the catheter remains occluded, and a fibrin cap or thrombus is confirmed by contrast injection, either catheter stripping or urokinase infusion therapy is warranted.

Air in line

1. Check the catheter for leakage by flushing well with normal saline.
2. Prefill injection cap with normal saline before attaching it to the catheter.
3. Check for loose connections.
4. Aspirate the air and irrigate the catheter with 10 mL normal saline to flush out any aspirated blood.
5. Flush and lock the catheter with heparin or normal saline.

Fluid leakage from catheter exit site

1. Infuse 10 mL of normal saline and observe for signs of fluid extravasation under the skin.
2. Obtain a dye study through the catheter to determine path of fluid flow.
3. Remove the catheter if a leak or transection is discovered inside the body.
4. If a leak is discovered in the catheter outside the body, repair it following the catheter repair procedure appropriate for the catheter type and the location of the damage.
5. If a fibrin sheath is encapsulating the catheter tip, instill urokinase (5,000 IU/mL) through the catheter into the fibrin capsule.

Catheter Damage

1. If the catheter is damaged, always fold the catheter between the patient and the damaged area and tape it together, or clamp the catheter between the patient and the damaged area with a smooth-edged atraumatic clamp.
2. Determine the site of damage and the size and type of catheter.
3. Refer to the catheter and adapter leg repair procedures to repair the damage. Use the appropriate size repair kit to insure a good repair.

Catheter and adapter leg repair

1. Assemble supplies included in the repair kit.
2. Clean the external segment of the catheter with antiseptic and gauze and place cleaned segment on a sterile drape.
3. Using sterile technique, put on sterile gloves, wipe powder from gloves with alcohol and 4 × 4 inch gauze, and create a sterile field with drapes.
4. Remove plunger from syringe barrel. Inject medical adhesive into syringe barrel, insert plunger, and attach blunt needle.
5. Reposition atraumatic clamp near the skin exit site.
6. Cut the external portion of the damaged catheter at a 90 degree angle just distal to the damaged area.
7. Insert the splice connector stent attached to the replacement catheter segment into the catheter lumen until the end of the replacement catheter tubing in ⅛ inch from the cut end of the catheter.
8. Dry space between catheter ends with a 4 × 4 inch gauze pad. Fill the ⅛-inch space with adhesive and approximate the catheter ends.
9. Use the syringe to apply adhesive onto the outside of the catheter around the spliced joint, covering an area about 1 inch overall length. Slide the splicing sleeve down and center it over the joint. Inject adhesive underneath each end of the splicing sleeve. Roll the splicing sleeve between fingers to distribute and extrude excess adhesive. Wipe away excess adhesive.
10. Sterile field no longer needed.
11. Remove clamp and gently fill catheter with heparin.
12. Fasten catheter repair joint to splint (application sticks or tongue blade) with tape. If necessary, the catheter may be used for infusion after 4 hours. The joint will not achieve full mechanical strength for 48 hours, at which time the splint may be removed.

Adapted from Paplham P. Post-procedural care of central venous catheters. *Semin Intervent Radiol* 1998; 15:297–303.

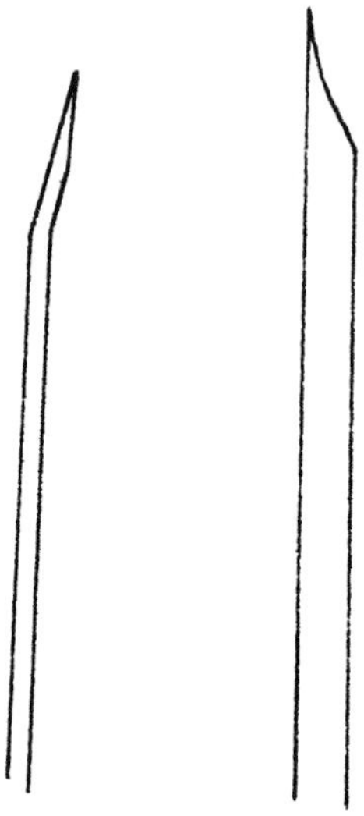

FIG. 10.1. Non-coring needle (left) and standard needle (right). Note the protected hole in the non-coring needle.

a standard cannula is used (Fig. 10.2). Although not as commonly used as the typical port system with a silicone septum, care providers should be aware that this type of port is commercially available and patients may present with such an implantable system.

Guidelines for accessing standard ports for both blood draws and infusion therapy are given in Table 10.2.

Care of the Incision or Catheter Insertion Site

Postprocedural care of the incision site for implantable devices depends in large part on the type of closure performed. In many instances, the skin may be closed with either subcuticular sutures or with adhesives; in either of these instances, there will be no external sutures to be cared for or removed following the implantation procedure. The routine at my institution is to keep the incision site clean and dry for 7 days. The dressing covering the incision site is changed every other day until day 7; dressing changes for port incisions do not require skin cleansing or topical ointment placement. The patient instead is directed simply to remove the old dressing and to place a new

dressing over the incision. After 7 days, the patient presents for a routine postprocedure follow-up visit. Assuming the incision looks healed, the dressing is removed and any external sutures are removed. Once the wound has adequately healed and sutures are removed, no dressing is required over the incision. It is important to remember to evaluate the venipuncture site as well as the port incision, and to remove any external sutures over the venipuncture site on postprocedure day 7.

In contrast to the exit site care provided for implantable devices, the care required for external catheters tends to be more involved. In addition to changing the dressing every other day, the catheter exit site and adjacent catheter must be thoroughly cleaned and prepared prior to placement of a new dressing. Guidelines for external catheter exit site care are given in Table 10.3.

Numerous studies have compared the efficacy of dressing types placed over external catheters. Advantages are noted with both dressing types. Gauze and tape dressings, for instance, allow better air flow through them when compared with many transparent type dressings; this decreases the amount of fluid trapped underneath the dressing. Transparent dressings allow the caregiver to assess the catheter exit site without actually removing the dressing itself, thereby theoretically decreasing the risk of infection to the exit site by decreasing the amount of time the exit site is uncov-

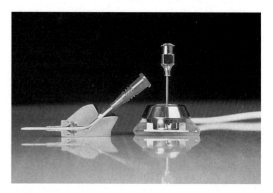

FIG. 10.2. The Cathlink system (left) allows access with a standard angiocatheter; a standard port system (right) must be accessed with a non-coring needle.

ered. By preventing the trapping of fluid, semipermeable transparent dressings (e.g., Opsite, Smith and Nephew, Massilon, OH, U.S.A.) may reduce the risk of exit site-related infections (3). Additional prospective studies are needed to further evaluate this dressing type.

A number of studies have been performed that have evaluated dressing types used for tunneled VAD (3,5–7). In an investigation by Conly et al., the authors concluded that the risk of catheter-related sepsis, local infection, and insertion site colonization were all decreased by using gauze and tape dressings as opposed to transparent dressings (3). In a more recent study of 101 bone marrow transplant patients, Brandt et al. compared gauze dressings changed every day with permeable transparent dressings changed every week (5). No statistically significant difference associated with catheter-related infections was found between the two groups, but costs associated with dressing changes in the transparent dressing group were calculated at just over one third the cost for the gauze and tape dressing group. Similar results have been achieved by other investigators (6,7).

The efficacy of using either polymicrobial or povidone-iodine ointments at the catheter exit site for external catheters is controversial. Although some studies have indicated a benefit to using the ointments (8), other studies have suggested no significant protective benefit by using the ointments routinely (9). Interestingly, a study by Flowers et al. concluded that the large number of catheter exit site contaminations due to *Candida albicans* were due at least in part to the administration of polymicrobial ointment to the exit sites (10). Flowers et al. suggested that because the polymicrobial ointment was not fungicidal, the *Candida* species were able to grow relatively unhindered by competition from other bacterial species. Further studies are necessary to confirm these findings.

Catheter Flushes

The catheter type, the indication for catheter flushes, and the occurrence of previous catheter-related complications determine the type and frequency of catheter flushes. General procedures for implantable and tunneled device flushes are given in Tables 10.2 and 10.3, respectively.

Most open-ended catheters (e.g., Hickman type) require flushing at least once a day; it is our routine to flush such catheters with a heparinized saline solution (10 U heparin per mL). Conversely, due to the slit valve located at the tip of close-ended catheters (e.g., Groshong type), these catheters may be flushed less frequently; in addition, they may be flushed with a simple saline solution. It is for this latter reason that a patient with either an allergy to heparin or with heparin-induced thrombocytopenia may benefit from placement of a closed-tip catheter.

Flushing catheters with antibiotic solutions has been performed in an attempt to decrease the incidence of delayed infectious complications. In the majority of investigations, catheter flushes were performed with either vancomycin alone or vancomycin in combination with heparin (12,11–16). In one investigation, tunneled central VADs placed in pediatric patients with hematologic malignancies were randomized to receive flushes with either heparin or flushes with a heparin-vancomycin solution (16). Bacteremia attributable to luminal colonization, as well as the time to the first episode of bacteremia, were both decreased in the group undergoing prophylactic antibiotic flushes. The cost effectiveness of such flushes was not assessed. Other investigators have demonstrated similarly successful results when using antibiotic prophylaxis (13–15,17). Conversely, multiple investigations have demonstrated no improvement in outcomes when using antibiotic prophylaxis (11,12). The efficacy of prophylactic antibiotic flushes in the prevention of catheter-related bacteremia remains open to debate; the cost effectiveness of such prophylaxis has not been completely addressed.

The practice of using thrombolytic agents for prophylaxis has been addressed in both implantable devices as well as tunneled catheters (18,19). In a study evaluating implantable port devices, a significant improvement in the incidence of catheter occlusions as well as infectious complications was noted when routine monthly flushes were performed with urokinase instead of heparinized saline (19). In a separate study, the number of delayed catheter complications noted in tunneled VADs also significantly decreased when prophylactic urokinase was given on a weekly basis (17% vs. ?% in the heparin control group) (18). The cost effectiveness of prophylactic thrombolytic flushes is still unanswered, and agents other than urokinase have not been individually assessed.

CONCLUSIONS

The role of the radiologist in the care of VADs continues to grow. In addition to placement of the device, the radiologist should be intrinsically involved in the decision on which type of device to place and when to place it, routine postprocedure care of such devices, and management of the complications associated with VADs. In order to provide the best quality of care to patients with VADs, it is essential to become familiar with the routine practices of VAD care in any given institution and to provide input into what those routine procedures should entail.

REFERENCES

1. Faubion WC, Wesley JR, Khalidi N, et al. Total parental nutrition catheters sepsis: impact of the team approach. *J Parenter Enter Nutr* 1986;10:642–645.
2. Raad II, Luna M, Khalil SM, et al. The relationship between the thrombotic and infectious complications of central venous catheters. *JAMA* 1994;271:1014–1016.
3. Conly JM, Grieves K, Peters B. A prospective, randomized study comparing transparent and dry gauze dressings for central venous catheters. *J Infect Dis* 1989;159:310–319.
4. Paplham P. Post-procedural care of central venous catheters. *Semin Intervent Radiol* 1998;15:297–303.
5. Brandt B, DePalma J, Irwin M, et al. Comparison of central venous catheter dressings in bone marrow transplant recipients. *Oncol Nurs Forum* 1996;23:829– 836.
6. Shivan JC, McGuire D, Freedman S, et al. A comparison of transparent adherent and dry sterile gauze dressings for long-term central catheters in patients undergoing bone marrow transplant. *Oncol Nurs Forum* 1991; 18:1349–1356.
7. Reynolds MG, Tebbs SE, Elliott TS. Do dressings with increased permeability reduce the incidence of central venous catheter related sepsis? *Intens Crit Care Nurs* 1997;13:26–29.
8. Levin A, Mason AJ, Jindal KK, et al. Prevention of hemodialysis subclavian catheter infections by topical povidone-iodine. *Kidney Int* 1991;40:934.
9. Maki DG, Band JD. A comparative study of polymicrobial and iodophor ointments in the prevention of vascular catheter-related infections. *Am J Med* 1981;70:739– 744.
10. Flowers RG, Schwenzer KJ, Kopel RF, et al. Efficacy of an attachable subcutaneous cuff for the prevention of intravascular catheter-related infection. A randomized, controlled trial. *JAMA* 1989;261:878–883.
11. Rackoff WR, Weiman JM, Jakobowski D, et al. A randomized, controlled trial of the efficacy of a heparin and vancomycin solution in preventing central venous catheter infections in children. *J Pediatr* 1995;127: 147–151.
12. Ranson MR, Oppenheim BA, Jackson A, et al. Double-blind placebo controlled study of vancomycin prophylaxis for central venous catheter insertion in cancer patients. *J Hosp Infect* 1990;15:95–102.
13. Carratala J, Niubo J, Fernandez-Sevilla A, et al. Randomized, double-blind trial of an antibiotic-lock technique for prevention of gram-positive central venous catheter-related infection in neutropenic patients with cancer. *Antimicrob Agents Chemother* 1999;43:2200– 2204.
14. Barriga FJ, Varas M, Potin M, et al. Efficacy of a vancomycin solution to prevent bacteremia associated with an indwelling central venous catheter in neutropenic and non-neutropenic cancer patients. *Me Pediatr Oncol* 1997;28:196–200.
15. Ocete E, Ruiz-Extremera A, Goicoechea A, et al. Low-dosage prophylactic vancomycin in central-venous catheters for neonates. *Early Hum Dev* 1998;53 (suppl):181–186.
16. Schwartz C, Henrickson KJ, Roghmann K, et al. Prevention of bacteremia attributed to luminal colonization of tunneled central venous catheters with vancomycin-susceptible organisms. *J Clin Oncol* 1990;8: 1591–1597.
17. Henrickson KJ, Axtell RA, Hoover SM, et al. Prevention of central venous catheter-related infections and thrombotic events in immunocompromised children by the use of vancomycin/ciprofloxacin/heparin flush solution: a randomized, multicenter, double-blind trial. *J Clin Oncol* 2000;18:1269–1278.
18. Ray CE, Sheroy S, McCarthy P, Broderick K, Kaufman J. Weekly prophylactic urokinase installation in tunneled central venous access devices. *J Vasc Intervent Radiol* 1999;10:1330–1334.
19. Fraschini G, Becker M, Bruso P, et al. Comparative trial of urokinase vs. heparin as prophylaxis for central venous ports. Presented at the 27th Annual Meeting of the American Society of Clinical Oncology. May 19–21, 1991, Houston, TX.

Central Venous Access
Edited by Charles E. Ray, Jr.
Lippincott Williams & Wilkins, Philadelphia © 2001.

11

Central Venous Access Device Placement in Pediatric Patients

Roger K. Harned II, MD

Department of Radiology, The Children's Hospital;
University of Colorado Health Sciences Center, Denver, Colorado 80218

It can be argued that placement of a venous access device (VAD) is no different in a child than it is in an adult. A patient with difficult access requires long-term or centrally administered intravenous (IV) medication, after which the appropriate device is selected and the route for insertion evaluated. The vein is imaged and accessed, and the device is implanted. Provision is made for postprocedure care of the chosen device. The reality is that successfully completing each of these steps requires addressing an additional set of problems that is unique to the pediatric population.

Patient size is the most obvious confounding factor—from the premature neonate to the bulky teenager. Special skills must be developed in order to consistently access the very small veins found in the young. One must be familiar with the small adult VADs that can be used in children as well as with some specific pediatric devices. Choice of which VAD to place will be influenced by the size and maturity of the patient in addition to their clinical needs.

One unique problem in children is the increased risk of dislodgment or migration due to growth. These catheters can be relatively short, and the tip position changes, sometimes rapidly, with the natural growth of the patient. Serial radiographs to evaluate tip position can be obtained at regular intervals until the patient has reached adult height. In young children undergoing rapid growth spurts, this may require surveillance as frequently as every 3 months (1).

Children are also much more likely than adults to require sedation for a VAD placement procedure. The necessary use of small veins requires absolute stillness on the part of the patient for successful access under imaging guidance. Preteenage children are frightened and usually unreasonable. For the patient's comfort and the success of the procedure, the operator must be familiar with a protocol for deeply sedating children in this age group. Local anesthesia with light sedation is adequate only in older patients.

Finally, the curious or uncooperative child must not be allowed to negate the hard work of VAD placement. Thorough and imaginative dressing and fixation of the VAD is necessary. Parents must be educated and willing allies in the preservation of venous access once it is successfully attained.

SEDATION

Success in obtaining pediatric venous access requires a well developed plan for keeping the child comfortable and still. Although soft restraints and papoose-type devices may immobilize a small patient for conventional radiographs or fluoroscopic examinations, they are not adequate for obtaining vascular access. The majority of patients under 10 years of age need some form of sedation to remain immobile for the procedure. Older children may tolerate holding still with local anesthesia alone. However, many will be referred to interventional radiology after multiple failed attempts at peripheral IV access or are long-term patients with cancer or cystic fibrosis who would simply rather not feel another needle.

Sedation protocols used when treating a pediatric patient vary greatly. An informal poll of interventional radiologists attending a sedation workshop given by the author at the 1999 Society for Cardiovascular and Interventional Radiology (San Diego, CA) found a few practices that relied almost exclusively on general anesthesia administered by an anesthesiologist whenever a pediatric case was performed. At the other end of the spectrum was at least one practice that routinely administered intravenous propofol, a sedative limited to use by anesthesiologists at many institutions. In our practice, less than 1% of the vascular access patients require general anesthesia. Other large pediatric centers have reported general anesthesia rates as high as 5% (2). Older or more stoic children who can tolerate catheter placement with local anesthesia alone account for 10% of our patients. Between these two extremes fall the large majority of pediatric patients who can be managed with IV sedation.

Intravenous sedation in pediatric practice cannot be equated with the "conscious sedation" that is usually effective in adults. The state of consciousness necessary to immobilize an infant or uncomfortable toddler better fits the designation of "deep sedation." In accordance with the published guidelines of the American Academy of Pediatrics, these children must be cared for as though under general anesthesia (3). To this end, our interventional suite has a crash cart equipped with child-sized resuscitation equipment and medication doses. We employ a nurse skilled in sedation to administer medication and monitor the patient. This nurse's primary responsibility is the patient, and this means that a second nurse or radiologic technologist must be available to assist the physician as needed during the procedure. Continuous pulse oximetry and electrocardiographic and respiratory rate monitoring are used along with blood pressure monitoring every 5 minutes.

Patient preparation for sedation includes a directed history and physical performed by the nurse administering sedation. Specifically, the patient's current medical condition, medications, allergies, and previous experience with sedation are assessed. The heart and airway are examined. An important piece of historical information to be obtained is the time of last oral ingestion. Although guidelines for fasting vary by institution, a recent literature review recommended waiting 2 to 3 hours following clear liquid ingestion and 4 to 8 hours for solid foods (4). At our institution, for interventional and diagnostic radiologic procedures requiring sedation we have used a minimum of 2 hours for clear liquids and 4 hours for solid foods. This has been applied to over 1,000 examinations per year for the past 10 years with no adverse effect. There is also controversy over whether breast milk should be treated as a clear liquid or solid. Our current practice is to treat breast milk, but not formula, as a clear liquid and allow ingestion up to 2 hours prior to the procedure.

In all patients for whom there is adequate lead time, we place a topical anesthetic at the anticipated site of percutaneous access. We have found this to be advantageous in several ways. Our agent of choice has been EMLA cream (lidocaine 2.5% and prilocaine 2.5%; AstraZeneca, Wilmington, DE, U.S.A.). EMLA cream must be applied 1 hour prior to the procedure in order to achieve adequate dermal analgesia. This requires a technologist or nurse to visit the patient prior to arrival in the radiology department. When applying the cream, this representative of the interventional radiology group can answer questions about the upcoming procedure and perhaps alleviate some apprehension on the part of parent or child. The proactive placement of a painless local anesthetic can be encouraging to a scared child, particularly when it can be demonstrated that the skin is numb right before starting the procedure. Finally, the patient can be evaluated for appropriate sedation planning. It is not unusual for our nurse returning from a patient's room to recommend a different level of sedation than that suggested by the referring physician.

EMLA cream maintains its analgesic effect for up to 2 hours after removal. This allows for some flexibility in timing of the cream application to accommodate delays and changes in schedule. It is essential to have trained personnel familiar with your preferred percutaneous entry site for the selected VAD. The usual location of the basilic vein for peripherally inserted central catheters (PICCs) or the internal jugular vein for tunneled catheters can be accurately anesthetized with experience. In those cases of variant anatomy or venous occlusion, the presence of analgesia in the skin some distance away from the eventual percutaneous access site still can frequently allow placement of a subcutaneous wheal of lidocaine at the site by initially placing the needle through the EMLA-anesthetized skin. Our standard practice is to place EMLA cream on both arms for PICC placement to maximize the probability of obtaining analgesia over an adequate vein.

Our current protocol for IV sedative medications is given in Table 11.1. Ketamine hydrochloride (Ketalar, Parke-Davis, Morris Plains, NJ, U.S.A.) is not a sedative used in adult practices because of the frequency of emergent reactions. This type of reaction is rare in prepubescent children, and this medication's other effects make it nearly ideal for short procedures such as vascular access. Administration via IV and intramuscular (IM) routes can be equally effective. The onset of effect is under 1 minute when given IV and under 5 minutes when given IM. It provides a dissociative anesthetic effect

that lasts around 15 minutes per dose, as well as a direct analgesic effect for 30 minutes. Respiratory depression is mild, and ketamine does not cause loss of upper airway muscle tone, as do the benzodiazepines. Finally, it is an inexpensive medication with no special storage or preparation requirements.

In practice we prefer to administer ketamine IV because of the rapid onset of action and the lack of discomfort from IV injection. However, because our patients frequently come to us after all avenues of peripheral access have been exhausted, an IM injection may be the best or only option. We begin with 1 mg/kg IV or 2 mg/kg IM (Table 11.1). Regardless of the route chosen, ketamine is always administered with a single dose of atropine sulfate. The anticholinergic effect of this second medication counteracts the hypersalivation seen as one of the side effects of ketamine sedation; respiratory compromise is possible if this precaution is not taken. The same dose of ketamine without atropine is repeated as necessary to maintain sedation. We administer additional doses to a maximum agreed upon in our institutional protocol, although no well-defined maximum dose exists for this medication. For procedures that become prolonged, a supplemental dose of Versed (midazolam hydrochloride; Roche Laboratories, Nutley, NJ, U.S.A.) may be given. In our hands this regimen approaches the results published by Cotsen et al., who described successful completion of 100% of interventional radiologic procedures performed in

TABLE 11.1. *Intravenous sedation for vascular access device placement in children*

Patient age	Sedative agent	Dose	Maximum dose
0–10 years	Ketamine hydrochloride plus	1 mg/kg IV	5 mg/kg
	atropine sulfate	0.01 mg/kg IV	
	Ketamine hydrochloride plus	2 mg/kg IM	6 mg/kg
	atropine sulfate	0.01 mg/kg IM	
	Midazolam hydrochloride (in addition to ketamine)	0.05 mg/kg IV	
>10 years	Midazolam hydrochloride plus	0.1 mg/kg IV, up to 2 mg maximum/dose	10 mg
	fentanyl citrate	1 µg/kg IV up to 50 µg maximum/dose	3 µg/kg

IV, intravenously; IM, intramuscularly.

211 patients who were 3 days to 10 years of age (5).

For patients over 10 years of age, we use the same sedative medications in common use for adult patients undergoing interventional radiologic procedures. Versed and fentanyl citrate are the drugs of choice; as with most pediatric medications, they are given in aliquots based on the weight of the patient. For children weighing up to 20 kg, a 0.1-mg/kg dose of Versed is given. Above this weight, an initial dose of 2 mg of Versed is given followed by additional doses of the same amount until the desired level of sedation is reached. After the initial dose of Versed is infused, a 1 μg/kg dose of fentanyl is given up to a maximum of 50 μg. This dose of fentanyl is repeated up to two times as needed (Table 11.1).

Our use of any of these medications is mitigated by several factors. When a request for vascular access is made, the requesting physician is questioned about the need for sedation in the patient. As previously mentioned, it is the rare child under 10 years of age who will hold still for the duration of a procedure. The primary care physician is a valuable resource for identifying these patients. The recommendations of the sedating nurse after application of EMLA cream and initial physical assessment are also taken into consideration. A final consideration is the possible calming effect of having a parent at the bedside while placing the VAD. Our general policy is to treat the interventional suite like an operating room with limited access to parents. The one exception has been the child in urgent need of a PICC who has airway compromise or other contraindication to sedation. Rather than using general anesthesia for a short procedure, we explore the option of allowing a parent to stay with the child and "talk them through" the procedure performed with local anesthesia only. When a parent is a good and willing coach, this has been successful in our experience.

OBTAINING PERIPHERAL VENOUS ACCESS IN CHILDREN

After the pediatric patient is adequately sedated, the next challenge is to image and access

a vein. PICCs are the most frequently requested VAD at our hospital and provide the greatest challenge because of the smaller size of the peripheral veins. Adolescents that have grown to adult dimensions can be approached in much the same manner as adults, as discussed elsewhere in this book (see Chapter 9). It is the newborn, infant, toddler, and small-for-age older child that will have correspondingly small veins in their extremities. This small size presents a number of problems.

A pediatric VAD candidate that presents with a peripheral IV in the arm can be imaged using conventional contrast venography. However, because of the difficulty obtaining any venous access in a child, patients frequently present with an IV in a foot or scalp vein. Although this provides a means to administer sedation, it does not help to visualize the upper extremity venous anatomy. Rather than have our nurse attempt to place an arm IV where other nurses have failed and, in the process, waste valuable minutes of sedation time, we instead proceed to imaging the veins via ultrasonography. Real-time sonography with a high-frequency linear transducer is performed with a tourniquet in place. We prefer to place a PICC above the elbow because this allows free range of motion of that joint after placement, and the veins tend to be larger as they become more central. Therefore, the basilic, cephalic, and brachial veins are quickly scanned in the transverse plane in both arms, and the largest vein is selected for access.

The upper arm is scrubbed a full 360 degrees around the arm from shoulder to elbow. This allows access to multiple sites on the chosen vein as well as to veins that are a second choice if the initial vein cannot be accessed. A sterile tourniquet at the shoulder allows the operator rapid access should it become necessary to release pressure to allow passage of a guidewire or between attempts at needle placement.

Except in very large patients, our needle of choice is a 22-gauge, 25-mm sheathed needle such as those in general use for peripheral IV access. The JELCO (Johnson & Johnson Medical, Arlington, TX, U.S.A.) and Quik-Cath (Baxter Healthcare Corporation, Deerfield, IL, U.S.A.) needles have a very sharp tip for puncturing the skin, which makes it easier to puncture the vein under sonographic visualization. The short length of these IV catheters is ideal for working in the small spaces around arms; they are frequently shorter than the access needles packaged with adult PICC kits.

Sonographic guidance of a small needle into a vein that may not be much larger than the sheath diameter is a skill that requires much practice. We use the method described by Donaldson et al. (6). Many cases must be performed to master this technique, and the initial cases using sonographic guidance typically take significantly longer than those performed fluoroscopically. At our institution, in order to improve our ultrasonographic skill we preferentially used ultrasonography for PICC placement on larger children not requiring sedation until these examination times decreased. At that point we were able to successfully expand to offer sonographic guidance to all sizes of patients.

The key element to success is the placement of the transducer transversely along the short axis of the selected vein and the access needle (Fig. 11.1). This is counter to most people's experience with sonographically guided procedures in which the transducer is held along the long axis of the needle and target. Size-related factors in small children make this familiar approach suboptimal. First, a small arm will not

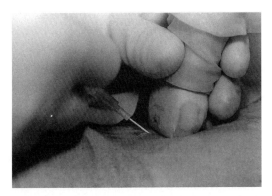

FIG. 11.1. The 22-gauge sheathed needle is aligned along the long axis of the basilic vein. The 10-MHz linear array transducer (encased in a sterile cover) is held perpendicular to the long axis of both vein and needle to allow a short axis image of the needle tip above the cross-section of the vein.

allow a linear transducer to be placed longitudinally and still leave adequate space above the elbow for needle placement. Second, the small vein being imaged can be smaller in diameter than the thickness of the ultrasonographic beam. Therefore, although still within the imaged section, a needle that appears to transfix the vein on a longitudinal image can actually be adjacent to it.

After the initial placement of the needle in the skin overlying the chosen vein, the transducer is slowly moved back and forth along the vein until the echogenic tip of the needle is identified (Fig. 11.2A). The needle and transducer are then slowly advanced such that the echogenic focus of the tip is seen to advance toward the vein and ultimately to efface its surface (Fig. 11.2B) The needle is then advanced until the tip is visible within the lumen (Fig. 11.2C). If possible, the sheath is advanced further into the lumen to ensure stability. At this point there is usually blood return through the needle. Occasionally the needle must be removed and the sheath gently retracted until free blood return is obtained. A 0.018-inch diameter wire is placed through the 22-gauge sheath and passed to the superior vena cava (SVC) to confirm that there is no venous obstruction along the planned path of the PICC.

Specific PICCs are discussed in a later section, but the maneuvers for placement are similar for all such devices. The 0.018-inch wire is used to place a peel-away sheath of appropriate size for the chosen catheter. With the small sheaths we find it helpful to dilate the tract to 0.5 to 1 French (Fr) size larger than the sheath to facilitate passage and avoid deformation of the very thin leading edge of the sheath. The guidewire tip is next placed at the junction of the SVC with the right atrium (RA). Our preferred method for transferring this length to the PICC is to lay the catheter on the skin overlying the sheath with the hub at the insertion site just as it will be when *in situ*. The wire is held firmly against the hub of the catheter and carefully withdrawn, maintaining the position against the catheter. The PICC is cut adjacent to the tip of the wire, ensuring a length equal to the distance to the SVC-RA junction. After insertion of the PICC through the sheath, the peel-away

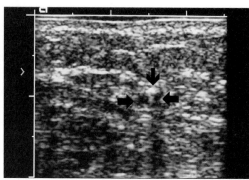

A

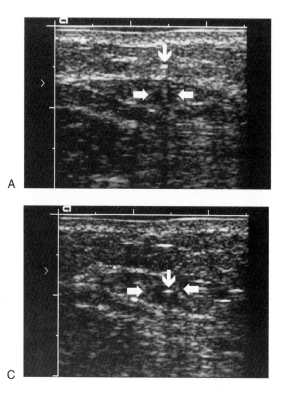

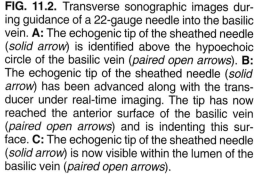

B

C

FIG. 11.2. Transverse sonographic images during guidance of a 22-gauge needle into the basilic vein. **A:** The echogenic tip of the sheathed needle (*solid arrow*) is identified above the hypoechoic circle of the basilic vein (*paired open arrows*). **B:** The echogenic tip of the sheathed needle (*solid arrow*) has been advanced along with the transducer under real-time imaging. The tip has now reached the anterior surface of the basilic vein (*paired open arrows*) and is indenting this surface. **C:** The echogenic tip of the sheathed needle (*solid arrow*) is now visible within the lumen of the basilic vein (*paired open arrows*).

sheath is removed and the tip position documented with a single-spot fluoroscopic image.

Children's veins do not always allow a straightforward insertion as described. Manipulation of a wire in a small venous lumen can result in frank injury and venous stenosis, or may lead to narrowing due to venospasm. In the acute setting these can be difficult to differentiate and even more frustrating to resolve. We take several steps to avoid this problem in the first place. As previously mentioned, gentle slight overdilation of the tract prior to placing the sheath can facilitate sheath passage into the vein. The very small sheaths can buckle at the leading edge and traumatize the vein. In very small children it is important not to advance the sheath its entire length into the vein. The tip can traumatize the vein at any slight bend (e.g., the junction of the axillary vein with the subclavian vein or the cephalic vein as it turns to its confluence with the subclavian vein). Careful maintenance of the sheath's tip in the straight portion of the accessed vein in the arm can minimize this problem. Wire choice also can have an ef-

fect. An angled Glidewire (Medi-Tech/Boston Scientific, Watertown, MA, U.S.A.) may facilitate navigation to the SVC, but its tip is stiffer than many wires, and the angle can increase irritation of the vascular endothelium. For this reason we use the Glidewire only when venography has demonstrated an area of vascular narrowing or tortuous collateral vessels that must be navigated. The Cope mandril wire (Cook Inc., Bloomington, IN, U.S.A.) or similar wire included in many PICC access kits has a soft, straight tip that in our experience causes less venospasm.

Using our method of placement we do not usually discover that venospasm has occurred until we attempt to place the PICC through the sheath. Although the original 0.018-inch wire apparently advanced easily to the SVC, the catheter may still buckle in the axillary or subclavian vein. Injection of contrast through the PICC shows narrowing or complete occlusion of the vein at this point. Unfortunately there are no universally successful treatments for venospasm, which may be due in part to the fact that all areas of venous stenosis are not due to venospasm but may instead be due to true vascular injury with perforation or dissection. Pharmacologic vasodilators such as nitroglycerin or papaverine given as a local infusion seldom alleviate the problem. We have had the most success by waiting 5 to 10 minutes to see if the venospasm resolves enough to allow passage of a wire. If a wire can bypass the narrowed segment, then gentle forward pressure is maintained on the PICC as it is passed over the wire. If venospasm or narrowing is recognized during initial passage of the wire to the SVC, then the wire is left in place rather than removing it to size the PICC. Instead, the catheter is draped on top of the patient along the course of the wire using fluoroscopic guidance and cut to the appropriate length. It is then advanced over the wire that has remained in place across the narrowed segment. When these simple measures fail, another site is selected for access rather than waste the remaining available sedation time.

Infants offer two alternative routes of peripheral access that are worth considering when venospasm, infection, or obstruction precludes use of the arm. Babies that are not yet mobile can tolerate a PICC placed in the femoral vein under fluoroscopic or sonographic guidance. The one caveat is that the inguinal crease is within the diapered area. To overcome the increased risk of infection we routinely tunnel the catheter to the mid-anterior thigh. Using this technique we have had no increase in infectious complications. The second alternative access route as described by Racadio et al. is through a scalp vein (7). A superficial temporal or posterior auricular vein is accessed under direct observation using a 22-gauge sheath needle system (Per-Q-Cath, Bard Access Systems, Salt Lake City, UT, U.S.A.). This system allows placement of a 2 Fr PICC. Under fluoroscopic guidance the catheter can be advanced to the internal or external jugular vein and, ultimately, the SVC. The reported success of this method is 48% placement in the SVC, with an additional 21% of catheters placed not in a central vein but in a final position that is deemed adequate for antibiotic therapy (7). This is well below the greater than 90% success rate of pediatric PICC placement in the arm (8–10), and for this reason scalp vein access is attempted only when other avenues have been exhausted.

Before completely abandoning hope of central venous access from a peripheral route, it is important to remember that tip position in a central vein is not an absolute requirement for every child referred for PICC placement. Patients referred for antibiotic therapy or infusion of another isotonic solution can be successfully treated with a PICC that does not reach the central veins. Indeed, the completion rate for antibiotic therapy and incidence of catheter failure has been shown to be similar for central and noncentral PICCs (11). Therefore, when we encounter venospasm or anatomic variants that do not allow the tip of the catheter to reach the central vessels, we consider the planned course of IV therapy and consult with the referring clinician. In many cases, a noncentral PICC is adequate; however, those patients requiring chemotherapy, inotropic medication, or other hyperosmolar preparations require another, nonperipheral approach to central access.

TUNNELED VENOUS ACCESS DEVICE PLACEMENT IN CHILDREN

With few exceptions, our technique for placement of tunneled catheters and implantable ports is not significantly different from that described for adults in other chapters of this book. Therefore, only those aspects pertinent to pediatric placement are emphasized here.

For tunneled catheters and ports placed in the chest, the internal jugular vein is our preferred vascular access site in all cases. This vein is large even in small children and allows placement of appropriately sized double-lumen catheters for long-term chemotherapy, total parenteral nutrition (TPN) or combinations of therapies. Access in the neck has a lower incidence of pneumothorax and hemothorax than does access via the subclavian veins. An attempt is first made to access the right internal jugular vein; if this approach is unsuccessful, the left internal jugular vein is used. It is rare to have to resort to the subclavian veins as a third option. Access is obtained under sonographic guidance in the transverse plane as previously described for PICC placement in the arm. One of the particular challenges in infants is the relatively short neck and large head. Use of the transducer on the short axis allows ample room for guiding a needle into the internal jugular vein of the mid-neck.

The access needle is exchanged for a peel-away sheath and a tunnel created from the lateral chest to the jugular insertion site using standard technique. If a port is being implanted, then a subcutaneous pocket is created at the proximal end of the tunnel. The catheter is drawn through the tunnel and cut to length by measuring against a wire that has been previously placed through the peel-away sheath into the SVC-RA junction. At this point there is some controversy regarding the relative risk of air embolism during the exchange of the catheter for the inner dilator of the peel-away sheath. Children present two challenges during this maneuver. Young children are sedated to the point that they are unable to cooperate with a request to exhale or suspend respiration. To complicate this, the young patient's respiratory rate is usually higher than that of an adult patient. The occurrence of air embolism in three patients led one large pediatric interventional group to recommend general anesthesia for all patients under 5 years of age undergoing placement of a central catheter via the internal jugular route (12). In this setting (i.e., a pharmacologically paralyzed patient), the anesthesiologist can suspend mechanical respiration and virtually ensure that negative intrathoracic pressure will not develop. At our institution, we continue to perform tunneled catheter placement under deep sedation in young children. Our method of minimizing the risk of air embolism during this critical step is that described by Kaye et al. (13). Adequate sedation must be administered to keep the patient comfortable such that they maintain a normal respiratory rate. The operator assesses the respiratory rhythm, and the dilator is retracted until nearly out but still sealing the sheath. As the patient exhales during the next respiration the dilator is completely removed and the catheter, which has been held

adjacent to the sheath, rapidly inserted. Like adults, older children can voluntarily hold their breath during this maneuver.

Ports have been implanted in the chest of patients as young as 23 days of age (14). Alternative sites also can be used, and peripherally implanted ports have been placed in children as young as 16 months (15). Our practice has been primarily in the placement of single- and double-lumen brachial ports in children over the age of 8 years. The technique is as described for adult patients, with our preferred site being above the elbow on the medial aspect of the arm.

A PICC placement technique also can be used for tunneled external port VADs. We have used this technique successfully in two patient populations. The first population is newborns with a hypoplastic left heart who have been referred for central venous access to be used for inotropic medication until a transplant heart becomes available. Because of the planned heart transplant, our referring cardiologists have preferred to avoid placement of catheters into the internal jugular and subclavian veins. One solution has been to place a single-lumen 3 Fr implantable catheter with a Dacron cuff (TPN Catheter, Cook) into the femoral vein and tunnel to the anterior thigh as described earlier in the section on peripheral access. A similar technique has been used successfully in the arms of two older patients with cystic fibrosis awaiting lung transplantation.

It is even possible to place high-flow VADs in the arm. Peripheral blood stem cell (PBSC) harvest is performed prior to transplantation in patients with certain childhood malignancies. These children frequently have an implanted VAD that has been used previously for chemotherapy. The tunneled catheter or port usually in place does not allow the blood flow rates necessary for the plasmapheresis performed during PBSC harvest. Rather than place a temporary internal jugular or subclavian vein catheter, we have put apheresis catheters in the basilic vein of the right arm (16). The catheter (Pediatric Hemo-Cath, MEDCOMP, Harleysville, PA, U.S.A.) is placed in the distal basilic vein high in the arm using the standard PICC technique

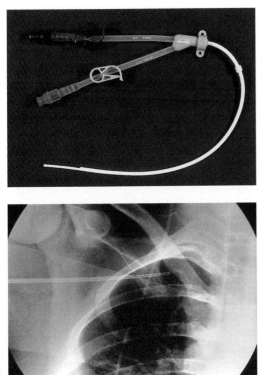

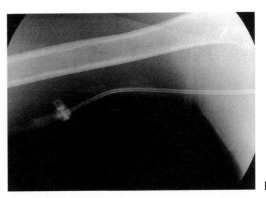

FIG. 11.3. Peripheral placement of a high-flow apheresis catheter. **A:** The 8 Fr, 24-cm apheresis catheter (Pediatric Hemo-Cath, MEDCOMP). **B:** Spot fluoroscopic image shows the position of the catheter in the upper arm. **C:** Because of the fixed catheter length, the tip position may be as proximal as the mid-subclavian vein in large children.

(Fig. 11.3). The Dacron cuff is placed just deep to the skin incision without creation of a true tunnel. This facilitates easy removal after the 1 to 7 days (mean 4) needed for plasmapheresis. Because the catheter is a fixed length of 24 cm, the tip position varies from the subclavian vein to the right atrium depending on the size of the child (Fig. 11.3). However, the stem cell harvests in children weighing more than 30 kg have compared favorably with those previously obtained using surgically placed internal jugular and subclavian catheters (16).

Children with complex or chronic clinical problems can require central venous access for long periods of time. In particular, those with malignancy or short bowel requiring ongoing TPN may have had multiple devices placed from an early age. Device failure or infection can require repeated removal and replacement. Many of these patients reach a point at which extremity, chest, and neck vessels no longer provide a direct route to the central vessels, but the need for venous access remains. Translum-

bar and transhepatic catheters as used in adult patients also have been placed successfully in children (1,17,18). The methods described elsewhere in this text can be applied to the pediatric patient.

PEDIATRIC VENOUS ACCESS DEVICES

The small veins in children can be difficult to image, challenging to access with a needle, and prone to injury and spasm. Once the needle and guidewire have successfully navigated the chosen vein, the next challenge is to insert an appropriately sized VAD. This can be both easier and more frustrating than choosing comparable devices for adult patients. It is easier because there are not nearly as many choices—therein lies the frustration as well. Pediatric VAD placement makes up a small percentage of most interventional practices not affiliated with a children's hospital. Manufacturers understandably supply catheters and ports in the sizes that are being used in large volumes. Fortunately the

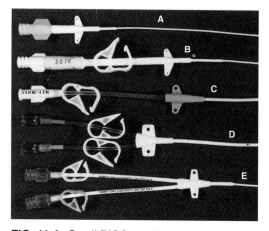

FIG. 11.4. Small PICCs available for placement in children. **A:** Cook 3 Fr silicone catheter with short hub and no clamp. **B:** Cook 3 Fr silicone catheter with regular hub and clamp. **C:** Cook 4 Fr polyurethane catheter. **D:** Medi-Tech 5 Fr Vaxcel dual-lumen catheter. **E:** SIMS Deltec 4 Fr dual-lumen catheter.

needs of small adults and the development of new designs and new materials that make devices smaller and more comfortable while maintaining longevity have provided some reasonable sizes of VADs for children.

We place more PICCs than any other VAD. Over 90% of those placed are the 3 Fr single-lumen catheter manufactured by Cook Inc. This soft silicone catheter is small enough for the neonate but provides adequate access for drug administration and blood draws even in the adolescent. It is available in two configurations, with and without a clamp (Fig. 11.4). Without the occluding clamp, the hub is shorter and better suited to the smaller patient's arms. Cook has recently introduced a polyurethane PICC in a 4 Fr size, which has a significantly larger lumen than the 3 Fr silicone PICC (Fig. 11.4). Four French is the maximum size we have had to place for adequate access using a single-lumen PICC.

Double-lumen PICCs are required when incompatible medications must be administered at the same time. Most dual-lumen silicone PICCs with an adequate inner lumen diameter are 7 Fr catheters, which are too large for most children under 30 kg. We have had good results with a 5 Fr double-lumen polyurethane catheter (Vaxcel dual-lumen PICC, Medi-Tech/Boston Scientific) (Fig. 11.4). This device can be placed in children as small as 10 to 15 kg when a vein of at least the catheter diameter can be visualized. A 4 Fr dual-lumen PICC has recently been introduced (SIMS Deltec, Inc., St. Paul, MN, U.S.A.) (Fig. 11.4). Our initial experience with this catheter has found no difference in occlusion rate when compared with the 5 Fr dual-lumen PICC. Dual-lumen 3.5 Fr catheters are available for umbilical venous catheterization, but our experience with these catheters has shown an unacceptable occlusion rate because of the extremely small lumens.

Implantable ports are available in almost innumerable variety. Innovative designs have larger or odd-sized diaphragms. Dual lumens can be side by side or in parallel. There is almost no way to keep up with the changes, and a great disadvantage of switching products with the introduction of every new port is that the health-care workers that access these ports may not become familiar with any one design. This is frustrating for patients and health-care workers alike. We believe in the use of a limited number of ports that offer the options our patient population needs. Using the same devices allows accurate long-term follow-up and enables identification of problems that might encourage evaluation of a new port designed to solve the problem.

We are asked to place single- and double-lumen ports, which may be placed in either the chest or arm depending on clinician and patient preference. Over the past 5 years we have come to stock just two ports to meet these needs. A chest port for a small child works equally well in the arm or chest of a teenager. Therefore, we have chosen the smallest and lowest profile ports that we have been able to find and use successfully. A light-weight material is preferable for patient comfort, although we recommend using a port with a radiopaque material marking the reservoir; this marker facilitates fluoroscopic needle placement in the event of difficulty accessing the septum by palpation alone. The single-lumen port we use is the Celsite Brachial Port (B. Braun Medical Inc., Beth-

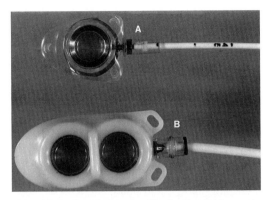

FIG. 11.5. Small, low-profile implantable ports available for placement in children. **A:** B. Braun Medical single-lumen Celsite Brachial Port. **B:** Bard SlimPort Rosenblatt dual-lumen port.

lehem, PA, U.S.A.) (Fig. 11.5). This is a low-weight device made of epoxy with a titanium reservoir. The locking device is a simple sliding sleeve that has not failed in our practice to date. The venous catheter is made of polyurethane with a 5 Fr diameter, which is the smallest currently manufactured port catheter. The dual-lumen port we have chosen to use is the SlimPort Rosenblatt dual port (Bard) (Fig. 11.5). The dual lumens are in parallel rather than in series, which facilitates placement in the upper arm of children weighing more than 30 kg and in the chest of any size child. The catheter is made of silicone with a 7 Fr diameter, which is the smallest manufactured catheter for a dual-lumen port. This is also a low-weight device made of plastic with titanium reservoirs.

Tunneled catheters with externalized ports are characterized by the Hickman or Broviac style devices. The basic design of a single- or multilumen catheter with a Dacron cuff meant to be placed in a subcutaneous tunnel does not seem to vary significantly from manufacturer to manufacturer. Our selection has been made on familiarity with a particular kit and the availability of small sizes. It is also essential that repair kits be available in all sizes of the catheter being placed because the external ports of tunneled catheters can crack or break following months of use. The ability to repair a cracked hub or more distal portion of a dual- or single-lumen catheter can significantly lengthen the life of the VAD in a child with limited access sites. The Cook line of TPN catheters has satisfied these requirements for us. The 3 Fr size is the smallest available and can be tunneled in the chest, leg, or arm as previously described. The 5F is as small as available in a dual-lumen style. Larger 7 and 9 Fr dual-lumen catheters are also manufactured in this line, and comprehensive repair kits for all sizes are available and effective.

VENOUS ACCESS DEVICE USE IN SPECIFIC CLINICAL SITUATIONS

The pediatric oncology patient requires months to years of vascular access for chemotherapy, antibiotics, blood products, and nutritional support. Additionally, they may become candidates for a bone marrow or stem cell transplant and need a high-flow VAD for PBSC harvest. Patterns of VAD selection in the oncology patient vary somewhat based on the bias of the referring clinicians. In general, it has been shown that the implantable port has a lower incidence of infection, accidental dislodgment, and catheter breakage when compared with the tunneled Hickman or Broviac catheter (19,20). Therefore, we encourage the use of totally implanted ports in all oncology patients. However, our pediatric oncology group continues to prefer the tunneled catheters in some specific situations. For instance, because of complex therapeutic protocols and prolonged hospital stays, patients with acute myelogenous leukemia, acute lymphoblastic leukemia with planned bone marrow transplantation, high-grade brain tumors, and stage IV neuroblastoma receive a double-lumen tunneled catheter. Patients with a low-grade solid tumor such as stage I or II Wilms tumor, rhabdomyosarcoma, or retinoblastoma can be managed with a single-lumen port. The remainder receive a double-lumen implantable port for primary therapy. Neither the externalized catheter nor the implantable port provide adequate flow for PBSC harvest. In the case of a child with one of these devices being referred for plasmapheresis, a peripheral 8 Fr apheresis catheter can be placed as previously described. This has been effective in patients over 30 kg (16). Smaller patients may require short-term placement of an apheresis catheter via the internal jugular vein.

Children with cystic fibrosis are prone to repeated respiratory infections requiring IV antibiotic therapy. These exacerbations can become more frequent as the patient gets older or as their pulmonary function worsens. In general, children under the age of 10 years present infrequently for IV therapy; when they do, they have relatively normal venous anatomy facilitating PICC placement on the floor or by the interventional radiologist. Many can even be managed by peripheral IV administration of medications. With frequent PICC placement or use of potentially sclerosant medications through peripheral IV catheters over several years, there is increased potential for venous stenosis or occlusion. When our cystic fibrosis patients begin to present more frequently than every 6 months for IV therapy, or caregivers have increasing difficulty finding adequate venous access for a PICC, we encourage them to consider placement of an implantable port. This is an idea that we try to introduce every time that we place a PICC in this patient population so that they can consider it in the coming months to years prior to their next presentation. It is not uncommon for older children thus prepared to decide on their own that an implantable port would be preferable to repeated and increasingly more difficult PICC placement. The usual antibiotic therapy requires only a single-lumen device, and most of the older cystic fibrosis patients who meet our criteria for port placement are older and prefer placement in the upper arm. This is cosmetically better and avoids discomfort from a chest port placed underneath the percussion vests used by some for respiratory therapy. At least one study has found a high complication rate in this population already prone to infection (21). Therefore, we do not encourage use of a port until the criteria described above have been met.

The neonate/infant under 10 kg is a challenge for short- or long-term venous access. Our smallest reliable VADs are 3 Fr, and we have found that, if a peripheral vein can be imaged

and accessed, then one of these catheters can be introduced. A simple 3 Fr PICC suffices for most applications requiring a few weeks of IV therapy. As mentioned in the section on preferred catheters, the Cook 3 Fr PICC without a clamp has a short hub that better fits the short upper arm of small patients.

POSTPROCEDURE CARE

All VADs are prone to the problems of infection, thrombosis, and dislodgment. The basics of regular catheter flushing with heparin, thrombolytics, and antibiotic therapy discussed in Chapter 10 apply to children as well. Catheter dislodgment, however, is an additional challenge in small patients who have no understanding in the first place of why they need the uncomfortable or clumsy device implanted in their chest or arm. Children do not voluntarily limit activity, particularly as they begin to recover from the condition that originally required the VAD. Babies cannot communicate the fact that a device is being pulled on before its short length is completely out. And, finally, tiny children in the intensive care unit may be a mass of multiple support devices clustered over a tiny surface area. The likelihood of an IV line being inadvertently removed while working on or transferring the patient is high. Therefore, it is imperative to take every precaution before and after the child leaves the interventional radiology suite to ensure that the device is secured.

The manner of catheter fixation to the skin is the first line of defense against accidental removal. All conventional PICCs are manufactured with a hub containing holes for sutures. Until 18 months ago we routinely used two interrupted stitches of Prolene (Ethicon Inc., Somerville, NJ, U.S.A.) to affix catheters. This is effective but has the disadvantage of a slightly increased infection risk from the presence of additional foreign material in the skin. The placement of these sutures also occurs at the end of the procedure as the patient is beginning to recover from the short-acting sedative medications we prefer. Because the catheter hub is proximal to the skin entry site, the sutures are usually placed through skin not origi-

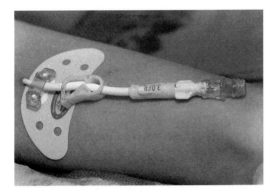

FIG. 11.6. StatLock PICC in place securing a 3 Fr PICC.

nally anesthetized. Either administering more local anesthetic or quick suturing without additional local anesthetic causes similar discomfort to the recovering patient. For these reasons we now use an adhesive device (StatLock PICC, Venetech International, Inc., San Diego, CA, U.S.A.) that holds as well as sutures and is quick and painless to apply. The catheter hub snaps onto two prongs on the adhesive pad that is then affixed to the skin (Fig. 11.6). Although Venetech manufactures a teddy bear-shaped device specifically for children, we have found that cutting the standard StatLock PICC down to a size to fit the patient's arm works very well in small patients. The single disadvantage to the adhesive device is that it must be replaced every 7 to 10 days of use because it eventually works free of the skin. Training of both our hospital and home care nurses has made this an easy and familiar task of routine PICC care.

The tunneled catheters we place do not have a hub for suturing and rely on the formation of fibrous tissue around the Dacron cuff to affix the catheter. This takes several days to develop, and for the previously discussed reasons, a child may not cooperate with allowing this to heal appropriately. At a minimum we close the small skin dermatotomy proximal to the cuff with a single Prolene suture. After knotting this stitch, the free ends of suture material are crisscrossed around the catheter and tied again. In very small children with short tunnels or active children who have demonstrated their ability to

dislodge a catheter, we take an additional step during placement. After the catheter has been drawn through the tunnel, the planned position of the cuff is determined. The catheter is withdrawn until the cuff is outside the body. A single stitch is placed through the skin at the planned cuff site and brought out through the tunnel at the proximal dermatotomy. The needle is passed superficially through the cuff without puncturing the catheter, then back through the tunnel, and out through the skin next to the original stitch. This is tightened as the catheter is drawn into position within the tunnel. Tying the suture at the skin provides additional retaining strength until the cuff elicits a firm fibrotic reaction. At that time the single loop of suture material can be ligated and removed.

Catheters placed in the arm are easily caught on clothing. Curious children also play with any object within their reach. No adhesive device or suture scheme stands up to strong or persistent tugging. It is therefore important to keep an arm catheter covered with the access port affixed and not flopping about. A loosely applied elastic wrap bandage can be applied, but this requires unwrapping for use and is bulky on small arms. We prefer a tubular elastic netting (Bandnet, Western Medical, Ltd., Tenafly, NJ, U.S.A.) that is available in multiple sizes. This netting slips over the catheter, holding it in place while still allowing access to the port for use (Fig. 11.7).

One of the frequently overlooked tools for successful postprocedure care of the pediatric VAD is the parent of the patient. In many cases the parent or primary caregiver is as likely as the child to inadvertently dislodge a catheter. The first step in preventing this is to assure that they are very familiar with the device. We show them a sample of the VAD to be placed and how it will be fixed to the skin. The parent is also instructed to dress the child in such a way as to minimize the patient's access to the site of the catheter. For babies, a "onesie" with snaps at the bottom will keep hands away from the chest and arms. Older infants and children do better with long-sleeve t-shirts. One piece pajamas with long sleeves are also helpful for preventing

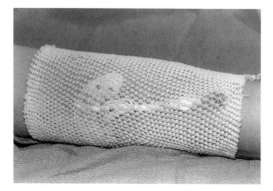

FIG. 11.7. Bandnet, in an appropriate size for the patient's arm, wraps and covers the PICC.

dislodgment or pulling while asleep. Finally, if the combination of Bandnet, StatLock or stitches, and parental care still fail, the educated parent can identify a catheter that is being retracted prior to complete loss of access. In these cases it may be possible to replace the device or place a new catheter slightly higher in the same vein. At the very least, a catheter still in the vein provides access for administration of intravenous sedation during placement of a new device.

REFERENCES

1. Azizkhan RG, Taylor LA, Jaques PF, et al. Percutaneous translumbar and transhepatic inferior vena caval catheters for prolonged vascular access in children. *J Pediatric Surg* 1992;27:165–169.
2. Donaldson JS, Norman JT, Morello FP, et al. Pediatric vascular access. *Semin Intervent Radiol* 1998;15:315–323.
3. Committee on Drugs, American Academy of Pediatrics. Guidelines for monitoring and management of pediatric patients during and after sedation for diagnostic and therapeutic procedures. *Pediatrics* 1992;89:1110–1114.
4. Krauss B, Green SM. Sedation and analgesia for procedures in children. *N Engl J Med* 2000;342:938–945.
5. Cotsen MR, Donaldson JS, Uejima T, et al. Efficacy of ketamine hydrochloride sedation in children for interventional radiologic procedures. *AJR* 1997;169:1019–1022.
6. Donaldson JS, Morello FP, Junewick JJ, et al. Peripherally inserted central venous catheters: US-guided vas-

cular access in pediatric patients. *Radiology* 1995;197:542–544.
7. Racadio JM, Johnson ND, Doellman DA. Peripherally inserted central venous catheters: success of scalp-vein access in infants and newborns. *Radiology* 1999;210:858–860.
8. Crowley JJ, Pereira JK, Harris LS, et al. Peripherally inserted central catheters: experience in 523 children. *Radiology* 1997;204:617–621.
9. Dubois J, Garel L, Tapiero B, et al. Peripherally inserted catheters in infants and children. *Radiology* 1997;204:622–626.
10. Chait PG, Ingram J, Phillips-Gordon C, et al. Peripherally inserted central catheters in children. *Radiology* 1995;197:775–778.
11. Thiagarajan RR, Bratton SL, Gettman T, et al. Efficacy of peripherally inserted central venous catheters placed in noncentral veins. *Arch Pediatr Adolesc Med* 1998;152:436–439.
12. Morello FP, Donaldson JS, Saker MC, et al. Air embolism during tunneled central catheter placement performed without general anesthesia in children: a potentially serious complication. *J Vasc Intervent Radiol* 1999;10:781–784.
13. Kaye R, Sane SS, Towbin RB. Pediatric Intervention: an update-part II. *JVIR* 2000;11:807–822.
14. Munro FD, Gillett PM, Wratten JC, et al. Totally implantable central venous access devices for paediatric oncology patients. *Med Pediatr Oncol* 1999;33:377–381.
15. Crowley JJ, Pereira JK, Harris LS, et al. Radiologic placement of long-term subcutaneous venous access ports in children. *AJR* 1998;171:257–260.
16. Harned RK II, Kelly SS, Foreman NK, et al. Peripheral placement of apheresis catheters in children: feasibility, safety, and efficacy in the collection of blood stem cells. *Radiology* 2001;218:294–298.
17. Robards JB, Jaques PF, Mauro MA, et al. Percutaneous translumbar inferior vena cava central line placement in a critically ill child. *Pediatr Radiol* 1989;19:140–141.
18. Malmgren N, Cwikiel W, Hochbergs P, et al. Percutaneous translumbar central venous catheter in infants and small children. *Pediatr Radiol* 1995;25:28–30.
19. Ingram J, Weitzman S, Greenberg ML, et al. Complications of indwelling venous access lines in the pediatric hematology patient: a prospective comparison of external venous catheters and subcutaneous ports. *Am J Pediatr Hematol Oncol* 1991;13:130–136.
20. Mirro J Jr, Rao BN, Kumar M, et al. A comparison of placement techniques and complications of externalized catheters and implantable port use in children with cancer. *J Pediatr Surg* 1990;25:120–124.
21. Deerojanawong J, Sawyer SM, Fink AM, et al. Totally implantable venous access devices in children with cystic fibrosis: incidence and type of complications. *Thorax* 1998;53:285–289.

Central Venous Access
Edited by Charles E. Ray, Jr.
Lippincott Williams & Wilkins, Philadelphia © 2001.

12

Alternative Routes of Central Venous Catheter Placement

John A. Kaufman, MD

Potter Interventional Institute, Portland, Oregon 97201

Patients that require chronic long-term central venous access are at risk for venous occlusion. Catheter-related central venous thrombosis is related to the underlying disease process, the access site, and device characteristics. The rate of catheter-related central venous thrombosis approaches 30% in some oncology populations (1). As access sites become occluded, the insertion of a secure, functional long-term central venous catheter becomes challenging. This chapter reviews techniques that have been devised for placement of central venous access devices in patients with limited access options.

PATIENT EVALUATION

Evaluation of the patient with limited access options should begin with a history, physical examination, and review of prior imaging studies and procedural records. Patients may have a history of multiple prior central venous lines, failed attempts at central access, infusion of sclerosing medications through peripheral intravenous lines, intravenous drug abuse, hemodialysis, plasmapheresis, or surgical interruption of the central veins. Specific questions should be asked regarding episodes of extremity swelling or hypercoaguable conditions. Additional risk factors include mediastinal masses, adenopathy, fibrosis, and radiation therapy. The location of previous central venous catheters should be determined. In addition, the presence and location of venous devices such as pacemakers, metallic stents, and vena cava filters

are important when planning venous access procedures (2).

On physical examination a swollen extremity with prominent superficial veins suggests central venous occlusion or stenosis (Table 12.1). Dilated veins should be traced from origin to termination if possible. Upper extremity veins that drain into abdominal wall veins are highly suggestive of superior vena cava (SVC) occlusion. Scars from previous central venous catheters, dialysis access, or other surgical procedures are important clues. The extent of a radiation portal can sometimes be determined from small permanent tattoos applied to guide therapy.

The amount of information that can be gleaned from prior imaging studies is always surprising (Fig. 12.1). The extent and age of an occlusion may be determined from serial examinations. Important venous anatomic variants or pathology in adjacent structures also may be discovered when a study is reviewed with a venous access procedure in mind.

When prior imaging studies are not available, a thorough evaluation of all possible alternative venous access routes should be performed. This evaluation should encompass both the peripheral and central veins. In particular, the status of the SVC and inferior vena cava (IVC) must be determined because they are the target vessels for most access strategies. Cross-sectional vascular imaging modalities may be required in addition to traditional venography.

Ultrasonography (US) can be used to determine patency of the upper and lower extremity

TABLE 12.1. *Important elements of patient history and examination*

History	Findings at physical examination
Prior lines	Scars from prior access
Phlebitis	Edema, dilated superficial veins, cords
Dialysis access	Scars, functioning or old shunts/fistulas
Radiation	Simulation tattoos, erythema
Hypercoaguable conditions	Adenopathy, surgical scars, cords

veins, as well as the deep veins of the neck. Gray-scale compression US can provide conclusive information regarding the presence of venous thrombosis (3,4). Doppler waveform analysis and color-flow imaging improves the ability to identify venous structures. Unfortunately, this modality is of limited utility when assessing the central thoracic and abdominal veins due to surrounding gas and the thickness of the overlying structures (4). Patency of the central veins can be inferred from normal gray-scale or Doppler waveforms in the peripheral vessels, but cross-sectional imaging with computed tomography (CT) or magnetic resonance imaging (MRI) is preferable.

Computed tomography and MRI can provide essential information when evaluating a patient for central venous occlusion or planning an alternative access (5,6). Contrast enhancement is crucial for venous imaging with CT, with attention to the route of access (i.e., the nonsymptomatic side when evaluating upper extremity veins) and acquisition of a delayed scan to visualize veins. Venous studies with MRI can be performed without contrast, although gadolinium-enhanced three-dimensional gradient-echo acquisitions are optimal. Both of these modalities produce data that can be postprocessed to better depict the venous structures. A major advantage of both CT and MRI is the ability to reliably visualize the deep central veins of the chest and abdomen. In addition, adjacent structures can be evaluated for anatomy and pathology.

Conventional venography remains the primary tool in the evaluation of the patient with limited venous access. This simple, safe procedure provides an enormous amount of information with regard to the nature and extent of occlusion. Perhaps most important, collateral pathways are preferentially filled, showing the point of central reconstitution and potential targets for achieving central venous access. Bilateral upper extremity venograms should be performed when evaluating the central thoracic veins. The jugular veins are not normally opacified with upper extremity injections, a recognized limitation of this technique; however, these veins are easily assessed via US.

PREVENTION OF CATHETER-RELATED CENTRAL VENOUS OCCLUSION

The ideal strategy for patients with limited central venous access is to avoid the problem in the first place. Reasonable attempts should be made to minimize venous trauma during punctures and insertion of catheters. The smallest diameter catheter possible should be placed, and a central location of the catheter tip should be ensured (Fig. 12.2). Administration of 1 mg of coumadin daily significantly decreases catheter-

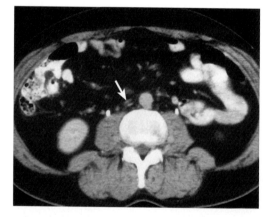

FIG. 12.1. Axial computed tomography (CT) image from a patient with an occluded superior vena cava. The patient was referred for a translumbar inferior vena cava (IVC) tunneled catheter. This CT scan, obtained for different reasons, was reviewed and revealed an obliterated infrarenal IVC (*arrow*). The patient underwent successful placement of a transhepatic catheter.

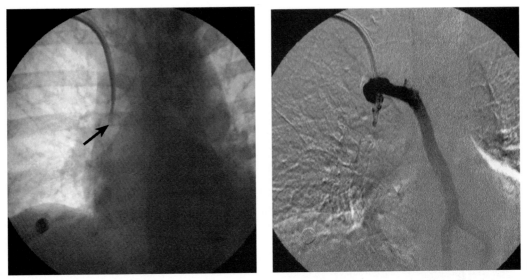

FIG. 12.2. Venous occlusion due to poor catheter tip position. Right subclavian dialysis catheter in a patient with bilateral internal and external jugular vein occlusions. **A:** Digital radiograph shows that the catheter tip (*arrow*) is in the superior vena cava (SVC), not the right atrium. **B:** Injection of contrast through the catheter shows thrombotic occlusion of the SVC with retrograde flow in the azygous system.

related central venous thrombosis in cancer patients (1). Prophylactic low-molecular-weight heparin (2,500 IU subcutaneously daily) also may prove beneficial (7). Long-term catheters coated with heparin or other medications are not yet commercially available in the United States.

ALTERNATIVE TECHNIQUES FOR CENTRAL VENOUS ACCESS

Alternative access procedures should be performed with the same strict attention to detail as conventional access procedures. Standard protocols for patient monitoring, conscious sedation, surgical scrub technique, and prophylactic antibiotics should be used. In most instances, alternative access procedures take longer and are more difficult than standard catheter placements, so an extra effort to maintain sterile technique is necessary.

Recanalization of Occluded Veins

Insertion of a long-term central venous access catheter through a vein that is already oc-

cluded is the ideal strategy in patients with limited access because no new veins are placed at risk (8). The objective of this approach is to successfully place a catheter, rather than recanalize the vein in the usual sense of relieving an obstruction. However, both goals can be accomplished simultaneously if desired (9). This approach uses conventional access routes and recanalization tools (Fig. 12.3). However, there is a risk that this approach will fail after much time and effort, resulting in conversion to a different approach. Therefore, before undertaking a recanalization procedure, the location, duration, and length of the occlusion, as well as the status of the collateral drainage pathways, should be considered.

The location of the occlusion determines the initial approach to gain access. In most circumstances, a patent segment of vein peripheral to the occluded segment is punctured. This provides a good target for the initial access, and a secure footing for catheter exchanges and venograms. Occasionally it may be necessary to directly puncture an occluded segment of vein. This approach works best for relatively re-

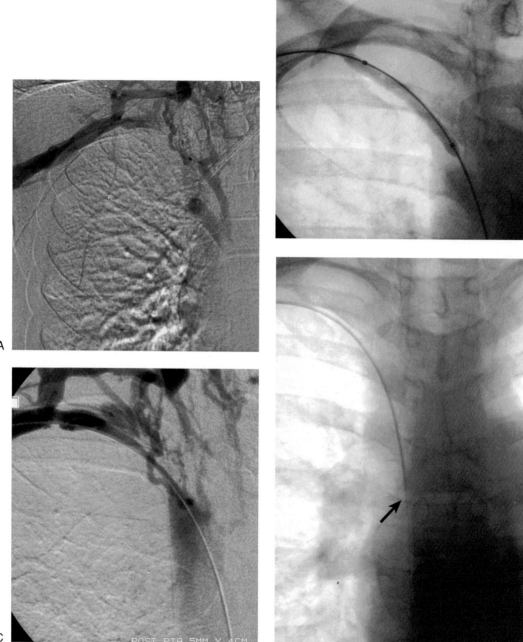

FIG. 12.3. Angioplasty of subclavian vein stenosis during insertion of a peripherally inserted central venous catheter. **A:** Arm venogram shows unexpected occlusion of the right subclavian vein at the junction with the internal jugular vein. Prominent collateral drainage is present. The patient was asymptomatic. **B:** The occlusion was crossed with a hydrophilic guidewire and dilated with a 5 × 4 cm balloon. **C:** Venogram showing the angioplasty result. The catheter was easily advanced over an 0.018-inch guidewire. **D:** Final image showing successful central placement of the catheter (*arrow*).

cent occlusions when the vein, distended by thrombus, is easily identified by US.

The duration of the occlusion is important when deciding to attempt recanalization. Chronic occlusions are difficult to cross with a guidewire, and catheters placed in such locations have a higher risk of ending up in an extravascular location than recent occlusions. This is particularly true with long occlusions. Recent occlusions of almost any length are less problematic, but without actually making an attempt, it may be difficult to predict how difficult it will be to cross the occlusion.

The status of collateral veins around an obstruction is a crucial consideration when contemplating recanalization procedures. Propagation of thrombus could occlude the collateral veins and lead to decompensation of the venous drainage. The risk is higher in patients with poorly developed collateral veins and an uncontrolled hypercoaguable diathesis. In this situation, a different strategy may be more appropriate. Occasionally a very enlarged collateral vein may offer a suitable conduit for a catheter (10).

Ultrasonography, venography, and CT can be used for the initial access. Micropuncture kits (Cook Inc., Bloomington, IN, U.S.A.) that allow puncture with a small-diameter needle and conversion to a larger system are invaluable for this approach. After initial access is obtained, an angled hydrophilic braided catheter such as an H-1 or C-2 with a tapered tip (Slip Cath, Cook) should be advanced to the site of obstruction. Injection of contrast may reveal a tiny residual lumen (the best possible case), or perhaps a small "nipple" that marks the former lumen. The occlusion can be probed with a 0.035- to 0.038-inch hydrophilic guidewire while using the angled catheter for additional directional control. A straight-tipped hydrophilic guidewire is sometimes preferable because an angled tip may select small branches as it is advanced. In difficult cases, progressively stiffer guidewires (including, as a last resort, the back end of an Amplatz guidewire) can be used as necessary to cross the lesion. Sharp recanalization with the needle from a transjugular intrahepatic

portosystemic shunt kit also has been described (11).

When antegrade attempts to cross an obstruction fail, a retrograde approach should be attempted if possible. An angled catheter is used in conjunction with a hydrophilic guidewire to cross the lesion, usually from a femoral access route. Larger, stiffer catheters such as 6 and 7 French (Fr) can be useful in the beginning, although 5 Fr hydrophilic catheters are frequently needed to cross the lesion. Long sheaths (40–60 cm) provide support for the catheter when working from a remote access, and exchange length guidewires are essential to avoid losing access during catheter exchanges. Once through the lesion, the retrograde guidewire may be snared through the antegrade access site. Ultimately an exchange length 0.035-inch Amplatz guidewire should be used to bridge the occlusion. Once achieved, this is a very secure situation, because the guidewire can be controlled from both ends during the introduction of dilators, sheaths, and catheters (body floss).

When the goal is limited to placing a catheter, dilatation with progressively large vascular dilators may be sufficient. For large devices, angioplasty of the entire tract with a 6- to 8-mm balloon results in a channel that will easily accept most catheters. A more durable recanalization is rarely necessary in this setting, but can be accomplished with placement of a stent immediately prior to catheter insertion. Prophylactic low-dose coumadin is strongly recommended to promote stent patency. Catheter-directed thrombolysis of an acute venous occlusion prior to placement of a long-term central venous access catheter may reduce the overall length of the lesion but significantly lengthens the duration of the procedure (10).

Once the occlusion has been successfully crossed and dilated, the introducer sheath for the catheter should be placed so that it is completely across the site of occlusion. This ensures that the catheter can be placed after the guidewire is removed. In some cases, the peel-away sheath provided with the access catheter may not be of sufficient length. If a longer peel-away sheath is not available, it may be necessary to place the catheter over a guidewire; in the latter case, predilation of the occlusion with an angioplasty balloon that is several millimeters larger in diameter than the catheter is helpful. Pinching the external end of the sheath tightly while loading the catheter onto the guidewire reduces (but does not exclude) the risk of air embolism and controls blood loss. Valved sheaths can be used when inserting ports that come with detached catheters. Occasionally a snare introduced from below may be used to pull a catheter through a recanalized vessel.

Translumbar Catheterization of the Inferior Vena Cava

First described in 1985, there is now substantial experience with translumbar placement of central venous catheters (12–17). Infection and occlusive IVC thrombosis rates are less than 5%, respectively, although catheter malfunction occurs more frequently (14,15). Long-term central venous access catheters of all types can be inserted with this approach, including large-bore dialysis and plasmapheresis catheters. Procedural complications such as retroperitoneal hematoma and arterial puncture have been reported (15). Catheter tip migration can occur due to patient movement, respiratory motion, or accidental dislodgment (16). Nevertheless, this access is straightforward, reliable, and durable (Table 12.2).

Patient evaluation for translumbar IVC catheters begins with evaluation of the skin of the lower back and abdomen of the right side. Open wounds, surgical drains, infection, or tumor involvement in these locations are contraindications to this approach. Because the catheter will be tunneled from the back to the anterior aspect of the lower abdomen, an unobstructed pathway must exist. In addition, patients must be able to lie in a decubitus or semi-prone position during the procedure. Review of cross-sectional imaging may reveal important information such as a left-sided IVC (17). An abdominal CT scan (with contrast) or a magnetic resonance venogram should be obtained prior to the procedure

TABLE 12.2. *Translumbar inferior vena cava central venous catheter placement*

1. Review prior abdominal imaging studies.
2. Examine skin of right lower back and abdomen.
3. Check coagulation studies, platelets.
4. Consider pigtail catheter in IVC via femoral approach.
5. Position patient left lateral decubitus or partially supine with right side elevated.
6. Wide skin preparation.
7. Use long 21-gauge micropuncture needle or translumbar aortography set.
8. Puncture just above right iliac crest 8-10 cm from midline.
9. Advance needle to just anterior to L2–3 to L3–4 interspace.
10. Aspirate as needle withdrawn until blood return.
11. Inject contrast to confirm position.
12. Use 0.035-inch Amplatz superstiff guidewire for dilatation.
13. Catheter tip should be above renal veins, preferably in right atrium.
14. Tunnel around curve of flank to lower chest/upper abdomen.
15. Locate port pockets over lower ribs anteriorly.

IVC, inferior vena cava.

if there is any question of caval patency, unusual anatomy, or retroperitoneal pathology. This is only necessary in the minority of patients.

There are relatively few contraindications to translumbar catheterization of the IVC. Coagulopathy should be corrected prior to the procedure, because puncture of lumbar arteries and the aorta can occur. The skin of the lower back and abdomen should be normal, without open or draining wounds. In patients with large abdominal aortic aneurysms, the IVC may be displaced and compressed, so that percutaneous access may not be feasible. This procedure can be performed successfully with an IVC filter in place (17).

When first attempting translumbar puncture of the IVC, it is helpful to insert a pigtail catheter into the IVC to serve as a target (Fig. 12.4). In addition, an initial cavogram can be obtained to confirm IVC anatomy and patency. When this approach is used, the femoral catheter is inserted with the patient in the supine position. After the catheter is positioned at the level of the L2–3 interspace, it is secured in place with

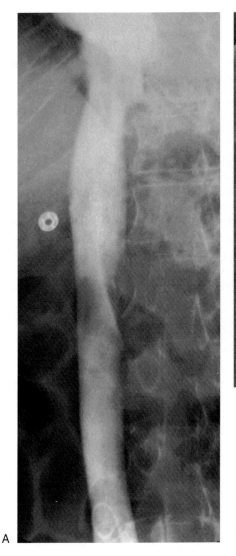

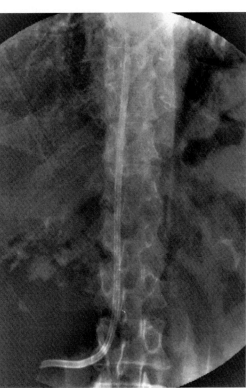

FIG. 12.4. Translumbar inferior vena cava (IVC) catheter. **A:** Cavogram prior to IVC puncture shows a patent vessel. **B:** Completion radiograph shows the catheter entering the IVC at the L3–4 interspace. The tip of the catheter is in the right atrium.

sterile adhesive (Tegaderm, 3M, Minneapolis, MN, U.S.A.) and connected to a continuous flush. Individuals experienced in translumbar IVC access may skip this step.

The patient is then turned to either the oblique prone (with the right side elevated) or the left lateral decubitus position (with a small towel roll between the left ribs and iliac crest to maintain a straight orientation of the lumbar spine). The sterile field extends from the table posteriorly across the flank and abdomen to the midline of the abdomen anteriorly, and from below the iliac crest to the nipples. The right arm is raised and placed across the chest in order to maximize the size of the field. A large area of preparation is required because the catheter will be tunneled from posterior to anterior. The patient is draped to allow access to both the right lower back and the right abdomen throughout the procedure. Fluoroscopy of the spine is then performed to localize the L2–3 interspace.

Translumbar puncture of the IVC is similar to translumbar puncture of the aorta in that the needle is inserted through the skin lateral and inferior to the final entry site into the vessel. The trajectory of the needle is cephalad and medial. The target entry level into the IVC is between the L2–3 and L3–4 vertebral interspaces; the usual location for the skin puncture is just over the right iliac crest 8 to 10 cm lateral to the lumbar spinous processes. After application of 1% to 2% xylocaine to the skin and subcutaneous tissues, a 1-cm incision is made with deep spreading of the soft tissues with a hemostat. Local anesthetic can be deposited along the anticipated path of the puncture using a spinal needle or the access needle itself. Patients feel pain as the retroperitoneal tissues are crossed with the access needle and dilators.

The choice of a particular access needle varies with the operator, but length adequate to reach the IVC is a common feature. Long microaccess kits with 21-gauge needles and 0.018-inch platinum-tipped guidewires are available, such as the Neff set (Cook) or AccuStick (Boston Scientific, Natick, MA, U.S.A.), but thin needles may be difficult to control in the tough retroperitoneal tissues. Alternatively, a large conventional translumbar aortography set may be used.

The needle is advanced toward the L2–3 vertebral body interspace just anterior to the spine. When using a C-arm, the tube can be angled so that the view is down the barrel of the needle, which greatly facilitates this process. If a catheter has already been placed in the IVC from a femoral approach, this can be used as the target. If the patient feels back pain as the needle is advanced, it can be treated with injection of additional small amounts of xylocaine. Deflection of the IVC catheter can be visualized just as the IVC is entered, or a faint click may be felt transmitted along the needle. A 20-mL syringe is then used to aspirate blood; if none is obtained, aspiration should continue as the needle is withdrawn until there is blood return. Once blood is aspirated, injection of a small amount of contrast will document the position of the needle tip. Arterial puncture is not a cause for alarm as long as it is recognized. The needle should be withdrawn and the angle of approach altered.

A soft-tipped guidewire appropriate for the access needle is advanced into the IVC, which is followed by placement of the coaxial dilator. If any question remains about the location or the identity of the vessel, contrast is injected again at this time. A medium-length (180-cm) 0.035-inch Amplatz super-stiff guidewire is then inserted; the tip of this guidewire should be advanced into the SVC if possible. Serial dilatation over this guidewire to the outer diameter of the peel-away sheath is then performed. Dilatation of the tract and IVC wall with a small angioplasty balloon (4–5 mm in diameter depending on the size of peel-away sheath) may be necessary in some patients.

The timing of catheter insertion depends on the type of device. For example, with detached ports the catheter is inserted at this point, whereas for one-piece devices the tunneling is completed first. In either case, when it is time to insert the catheter, a peel-away sheath is first inserted over the guidewire. This sheath must be long enough to provide secure access to the IVC after removal of the guidewire. When a relatively flat trajectory has been used to enter the IVC, the sheath may kink at the vessel once the dilator is removed. Preloading a hydrophilic guidewire into the catheter prior to insertion into the sheath is useful in this situation. The guidewire can usually be advanced through the kink, straightening the sheath enough to allow passage of the catheter. If the guidewire fails to straighten the kink, the sheath can be withdrawn slightly over the guidewire to reposition the kink in the tract. The peel-away sheath should be at least 1 Fr size larger than the catheter to minimize friction during the peel-away insertion.

The catheter tip should be positioned as high as possible in the IVC, preferably at the junction with the right atrium. At the very least, the catheter tip should be above the renal veins to take advantage of the high renal inflow.

The subcutaneous tunnel from the puncture site to the skin exit site or pocket is then anesthetized with 1% to 2% xylocaine. Long tunnels may be divided into one or two segments with small port-hole incisions. This is frequently necessary because the tunneling devices are rarely long or malleable enough to tunnel around the curve of the flank. Ports should be located over the inferior aspect of the anterior ribs to provide support during access. External catheters should exit the skin above the patient's beltline for comfort and ease of care. Routine flushing, skin closure techniques, and dressings should be used at the completion of the procedure.

Transhepatic Catheterization of the Inferior Vena Cava

Occlusion of both the SVC and infrarenal IVC occurs in a small number of patients. With few exceptions the intrahepatic portion of the IVC remains patent. Transhepatic central venous catheters can be placed through a hepatic vein or directly into the intrahepatic IVC (18,19). All types of catheters have been placed in this manner, including dialysis catheters (20). This approach has been successful in the adult and the pediatric population (21,22). In children, transhepatic access has been used for diagnostic and interventional procedures in addition to chronic venous access (23). In adults, the transhepatic approach for long-term central venous catheterization is usually reserved for patients with no other access options (Table 12.3).

The body of literature reporting on this approach is smaller than that with translumbar catheters, and is limited to some case reports and small series. In properly selected patients, this is a safe and durable method of access. Unique complications include early catheter dislodgment with bleeding from the hepatic tract and thrombosis of the hepatic vein around the catheter (24). Dislodgement occurs most often in active patients, presumably due to gradual retraction of the catheter during deep respiration. Contraindications include uncorrected coagulopathy, massive ascites, active hepatic or biliary infection, vascular hepatic tumors along the anticipated path of the catheter, and inability to puncture or tunnel through normal skin. Prior partial hepatectomy, a small vol-

TABLE 12.3. *Transhepatic central venous catheter placement*

1. Obtain cross-sectional imaging studies.
2. Examine skin of right flank and upper abdomen.
3. Check coagulation studies, platelets.
4. Position patient supine (right arm behind head for mid-axillary approach).
5. Wide skin preparation.
6. Select lateral intercostal (mid-axillary line) or anterior subcostal puncture.
7. Consider ultrasonographic guidance for subcostal puncture.
8. Use long 21-gauge micropuncture needle.
9. Do not cross midline with needle tip.
10. Target is intrahepatic IVC or middle hepatic vein (latter preferred in children).
11. Aspirate as needle is withdrawn until blood return.
12. Inject contrast to confirm location.
13. Use 0.035-inch Amplatz superstiff guidewire for dilatation (be careful of wire tip in heart).
14. Locate port pockets over lower anterior ribs.
15. Catheter tip should be in right atrium.

IVC, inferior vena cava.

ume of ascites, and polycystic liver disease are relative contraindications.

Direct puncture of the intrahepatic IVC provides the longest path through the hepatic parenchyma, which may help stabilize the catheter in patients with extensive diaphragmatic excursion during respiration. Puncture of a hepatic vein (usually the middle) results in a longer intravascular length of the catheter, an important consideration in children who may literally outgrow the catheter. This approach carries the risk of hepatic vein thrombosis, a complication that is usually asymptomatic as long as other hepatic veins are patent.

Patient evaluation consists of cross-sectional hepatic imaging, preferably a contrast-enhanced CT scan. The liver, hepatic veins, intrahepatic IVC, subphrenic space, and the perihepatic peritoneal cavity should be normal. Transhepatic placement of a central venous catheter should not be attempted without preprocedural cross-sectional imaging. The skin of the right upper quadrant should be free of infection and tumor.

The patient is placed in the supine position on the fluoroscopy table. When right lateral intercostal access is anticipated, the right arm is abducted to 90 degrees. For the anterior sub-costal approach, the arm can remain by the patient's side. The skin is prepared from the table on the right flank to the midline of the abdomen, and from the right iliac crest to the right nipple. The patient is draped so that the access site and anticipated skin exit or pocket site are accessible.

Lateral access is usually through the 10th or 11th interspace in the mid-axillary line, but fluoroscopy during inspiration and expiration is essential to determine the location of the pleural reflection. Local anesthetic is injected subcutaneously and over the top border of the rib. In most patients a 22-gauge, 1.5-inch hypodermic needle can be used to anesthetize the liver capsule. Through a 1-cm skin incision a microaccess needle is advanced over the top of the rib in a horizontal plane toward the spine. Respiration is suspended for this portion of the procedure, and the needle should not pass beyond the midline of the spine. Return of blood during withdrawal of the needle is followed by injection of contrast to identify the vessel. The entry site can be either the middle hepatic vein or the IVC. Ultrasonographic guidance is sometimes necessary, particularly when trying to puncture the middle hepatic vein.

A subcostal approach can be used when anterior access is desired. The planned entry site is the middle hepatic vein; the procedure is otherwise identical to the lateral intercostal approach. Routine ultrasonographic guidance is advised for a subcostal puncture.

Once venous access is obtained, a 0.018-inch platinum tipped guidewire is advanced into the right atrium. A coaxial dilator is then advanced into the IVC, and the guidewire exchanged for a standard-length 0.035-inch Amplatz super-stiff guidewire. Whenever possible, the tip of this guidewire should be positioned in the SVC to avoid atrial or ventricular dysrhythmias. Serial dilation over the guidewire allows insertion of the peel-away sheath, and ultimately the access catheter. The tip of the catheter should be just into the right atrium (Fig. 12.5).

The timing of insertion of the catheter depends on the type of device; one-piece catheters are inserted after tunneling, whereas catheters that are supplied detached from ports are inserted first, then tunneled back to the pocket. Whenever a difficult catheter insertion is anticipated, a hydrophilic guidewire should be preloaded into the catheter, or insertion over a guidewire should be considered. Standard-length peel-away sheaths may not be sufficient to reach the IVC in some patients, but this problem is not encountered as often as with translumbar catheters.

When tunneling the catheter, a small amount of redundancy in the subcutaneous tissue at the entry site helps prevent movement of the catheter tip with respiration. The degree of the catheter excursion with respiration can be assessed during the procedure by having the patient inhale and exhale deeply while observing with fluoroscopy. Catheters placed through a mid-axillary access are tunneled anteriorly in a manner similar to that for translumbar catheter insertion. Pockets for ports should be created over the lower anterior ribs to provide a firm target during access. Standard suture techniques, catheter flushing, dressings, and wound care should be used.

Removal of transhepatic catheters differs from other venous lines. The principle risk is intraperitoneal or subcapsular hemorrhage from an immature catheter track. Catheters that have been in place for several weeks have a well-developed fibrous tunnel that excludes the peritoneal space (although this may not be true in patients with ascites). Embolization of the track with gelfoam pledgets should be considered for acute removal of large diameter noninfected catheters (23). This can done by cutting down on the catheter at the puncture site, gaining control of the exposed catheter, transecting the catheter, placing a hydrophilic guidewire through the intravascular portion of the catheter, and exchanging the catheter for a sheath through which the gelfoam can be deposited.

Femoral Vein Central Venous Catheterization

Long-term central venous access via the femoral vein has been used for longer than the translumbar or transhepatic routes, but remains

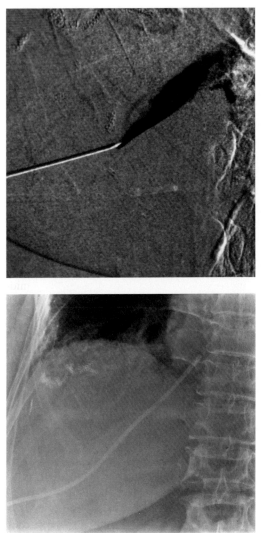

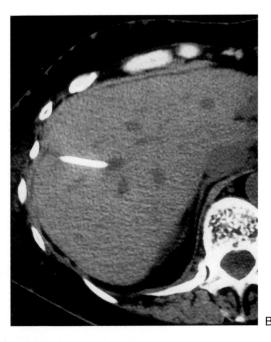

FIG. 12.5. Transhepatic cannulation of the IVC via the middle hepatic vein in a patient with occlusions of the superior and infrarenal inferior vena cavae. (Reprinted from Kaufman JA et al. Long-term central venous catheterization in patients with limited access. *AJR* 1996;167:1327–1333; with permission.) **A:** Digital subtraction venogram performed through the microaccess needle confirms puncture of a hepatic vein. **B:** Postprocedural computed tomography scan shows the catheter as it enters the middle hepatic vein. **C:** Postplacement chest radiograph shows the tip of the catheter in the right atrium. The course of the catheter conforms to that of the middle hepatic vein.

somewhat controversial (25–28). This access is commonly used in pediatric patients in the acute care setting, but less often in adults (29,30). All types of chronic access catheters have been placed through the femoral vein, including hemodialysis catheters (28).

Most patients who are candidates for the femoral approach could also have translumbar catheters. Advantages of femoral vein catheters are simplicity of access and easier tunneling (25–28). The disadvantages are the increased risk of iliofemoral vein thrombosis and infection that have been reported with these devices

(28,29). In one series of acute-care nontunneled femoral vein catheters in adults, the rate of ultrasonographically diagnosed femoral thrombosis was 25% (30). The reported rate of IVC and iliofemoral thrombosis has been much lower with tunneled access catheters, approaching 10% in some series (26,28). Most clinicians use the right common femoral vein for access, so there are no data reporting on side of access and risk of thrombosis. In addition, comprehensive surveillance for catheter-related venous thrombosis has not been routinely performed in most series, so the rate of asymptomatic thrombosis may actually be higher. A higher incidence of bacteremia has been reported with nontunneled catheters in comparison with tunneled devices (27). The documented infection rate with tunneled femoral dialysis catheters was 5.2/1,000 days in one report (28).

The status of the iliofemoral veins and IVC should be determined in patients undergoing femoral vein catheter placement whenever there is a past history of venous instrumentation, abdominal or pelvic masses, leg swelling, or thromboembolic disease. Compression ultrasonography of the common femoral vein with Doppler interrogation of femoral venous flow during deep respiration and Valsalva maneuver should be obtained as an initial study. A compressible common femoral vein with normal Doppler flow patterns implies a patent access site and central veins. Further evaluation with CT or magnetic resonance venography may be useful in cases with abnormal ultrasonographic results. The skin integrity in the inguinal region, upper thigh, and lower abdomen should be evaluated. Special note of the normal location of the patient's beltline should be made (Table 12.4).

Contraindications to the femoral venous approach include uncorrected coagulopathy, infection or other dermatologic conditions in the inguinal region, and open lower quadrant wounds. Prior episodes of iliofemoral deep venous thrombosis on the side of access is a potential contraindication because the patient may be at higher risk for a recurrent thrombosis with a catheter in place. However, presence of a vena cava filter is not a contraindication.

The patient should be positioned for a routine femoral venous puncture. The skin should be prepared laterally from the greater trochanter to the midline of the abdomen, and from the mid-thigh to anterior costal margin. In general, the right common femoral vein is preferred due to less iliac vein tortuosity and a theoretical lower risk of thrombosis. Compression of the left common iliac vein by the right common iliac artery may make catheter-related thrombosis more likely with left-sided approaches.

The common femoral vein is punctured in the normal location with either a microaccess

TABLE 12.4. *Femoral central venous catheter placement*

1. Review prior abdominal imaging studies.
2. Right common femoral vein access if possible.
3. Examine skin of groin, thigh and lower abdomen.
4. Check coagulation studies, platelets.
5. Position patient supine.
6. Wide skin preparation.
7. Puncture common femoral vein.
8. Consider ultrasonographic guidance.
9. Aspirated blood confirms location.
10. Inject contrast to confirm central patency if necessary.
11. Use 0.035-inch Amplatz superstiff guidewire for dilatation.
12. Position catheter tip in right atrium or as close as possible.
13. Tunnel onto thigh or lateral lower abdomen.
14. Use subcuticular closure groin incision.

needle or a standard angiographic needle. Should there be any question of venous patency or anatomy, contrast is injected through a dilator. A standard-length 0.035-inch Amplatz superstiff guidewire is inserted and serial dilation to the size of the introducer sheath is accomplished. The catheter is then inserted through a peel-away sheath, with the tip positioned as high as possible in the IVC (ideally at the cavoatrial junction). Long devices (sometimes 60 cm in length or more) are needed for the femoral venous approach. Sheath kinking is a rare problem with this access (Fig. 12.6).

Catheters can be tunneled either down the thigh or onto the abdomen (28). Good clinical results and patient acceptance have been reported with both. The advantage of having the skin exit site or port on the abdomen is that it can be located above the beltline, which simplifies access and care. Abdominal tunnels should swing laterally to ensure a gentle curve at the catheter insertion site.

The groin incision is closed with subcuticular sutures (such as 4–0 Dexon) to minimize the risk of infection. External sutures are difficult to keep clean in the groin and may provide a pathway for bacteria to enter the subcutaneous tissues. Otherwise, standard catheter flushing, wound care, and dressing protocols should be used. Prophylactic therapy with coumadin (1 mg daily) is suggested to prevent catheter-

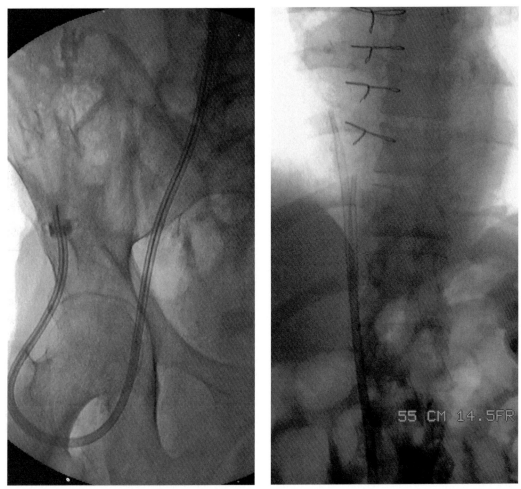

FIG. 12.6. Femoral vein hemodialysis catheter in a patient with obstruction of the superior vena cava due to multiple prior catheters. **A:** The catheter is tunneled superiorly and laterally. **B:** The catheter tip is in the right atrium.

related iliofemoral thrombosis. Thrombosis is treated with full anticoagulation in the same manner as conventional deep vein thrombosis, but the catheter should be left in place if possible. (28).

Catheterization of Collateral Veins

Enlarged upper extremity collateral veins can sometimes be successfully negotiated to permit central positioning of a catheter (10,31). This has been described as an entirely percutaneous technique, or in combination with surgery (32). Lower truncal collateral veins also have been used for alternative venous access (33). Experience with this approach is limited, with a number of case reports but no substantial series of patients in the literature. In general, these have been patients in whom other alternative access was not available, or in whom an enlarged collateral vein was serendipitously encountered during an access procedure that was then used.

Contrast venography is very useful when planning the procedure, because it allows the interventionalist to determine the quality of the collateral vein and the reconstituted central vein. Simultaneous bilateral upper extremity venograms, or direct injection of an enlarged

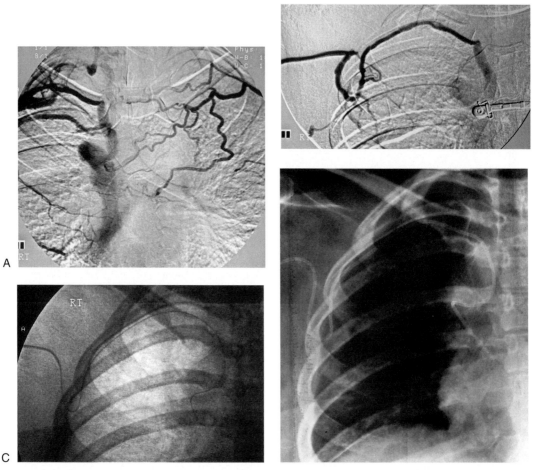

C   D

FIG. 12.7. Transcollateral catheter in a 27-year-old woman with Hodgkin disease who was referred for placement of an implantable venous access device. (Reprinted from Kaufman JA, Crenshaw WB, Kuter I, et al. Percutaneous placement of a central venous access device via an intercostal vein. *AJR* 1995;165:459–460; with permission.) **A:** Digital subtraction venogram of both upper extremities shows occlusion of the major central thoracic veins with the exception of the azygous vein and the infraazygous superior vena cava (SVC). **B:** Digital subtraction venogram of an injection into a right lateral chest wall vein. The right third intercostal vein is filled and drains into a patent azygous vein, and ultimately the SVC. **C:** Image showing the course of a hydrophilic guidewire used to negotiate the collateral vein to the SVC. **D:** Chest radiograph obtained after completion of the procedure shows position of the catheter. The catheter tip is in the SVC below the azygous arch.

superficial neck or chest vein, may be required (Fig. 12.7). Although CT and MRI may reveal more collateral veins than venography, they may not be usable due to size, location, tortuosity, or stenoses. Direct punctures of the intercostal and hemiazygous veins have been reported, as has catheterization of a chest wall collateral vein from the basilic vein to reach the intercostal veins (10,31,32). The full range of angiographic tools may be required for a successful procedure, including hydrophilic selective catheters and expensive torque-control guidewires. Catheter tips have been placed in the SVC or left within an enlarged azygous vein (31,32). An important consideration when attempting this approach is the status of other collateral veins, because catheter-induced thrombosis of a major or isolated draining vein may precipitate severe symptoms. This particular approach to venous access requires maximal creativity on the part of the interventionalist.

Miscellaneous and Surgical Approaches

Almost any vein in the body that ultimately drains centrally can be potentially used for percutaneous access. For example, insertion of 2 Fr peripherally inserted central venous catheters (PICC lines) through scalp veins in infants permitted central (SVC) placement in 48% of attempts in one report (34). Cannulation of small peripheral veins and negotiation into the central veins may require sophisticated angiographic tools, excellent imaging, small access devices, and (most important) lots of time. With the combined use of fluoroscopy and cross-sectional imaging it is possible to puncture veins that would be difficult to opacify from a peripheral access, such as gonadal veins. Whenever attempting a new or unusual approach, it is important to thoroughly review the patient's prior imaging studies as well as the relevant cross-sectional anatomy to avoid inadvertent puncture of adjacent structures.

Numerous surgical options have been described for alternative venous access. These include the ovarian, iliac, internal mammary, and azygous veins, and direct cannulation of the right atrium (35–39). Combined surgical and percutaneous techniques have been described to recanalize occluded central veins, but these have become less common following the development of current angiographic tools, imaging techniques, and radiologic interest in central venous access (40). Some of these approaches may now be feasible as wholly percutaneous techniques with newer tools and appropriate image guidance.

CONCLUSION

Prevention of catheter-related central venous occlusion would greatly reduce the need for the techniques described in this chapter. However, this goal will remain elusive in the near future.

Patients with limited options for long-term central venous access require careful evaluation of the available veins and access needs, thorough preprocedural planning, careful attention to detail during the procedure, and innovation. Successful catheter placement is of invaluable benefit, and often life saving, for these patients.

REFERENCES

1. Bern MM, Lokich JJ, Wallach SR, et al. Very low dose warfarin can prevent thrombosis in central venous catheters. A randomized prospective trial. *Ann Intern Med* 1990;112:423–428.
2. Spence LD, Gironta MG, Malde HM, et al. Acute upper extremity deep venous thrombosis: safety and effectiveness of superior vena caval filters. *Radiology* 1999; 210:53–58.
3. Fraser JD, Anderson DR. Deep venous thrombosis: recent advances and optimal investigation with US. *Radiology* 1999;211:9–24.
4. Passman MA, Criado E, Farber MA, et al. Efficacy of color flow duplex imaging for proximal upper extremity venous outflow obstruction in hemodialysis patients. *J Vasc Surg* 1998;28:869–875.
5. Qanadli SD, Hajjam ME, Bruckert F, et al. Helical CT phlebography of the superior vena cava: diagnosis and evaluation of venous obstruction. *AJR* 1999;172:1327–1333.
6. Li W, David V, Kaplan R, Edelman RR. Three-dimensional low dose gadolinium-enhanced peripheral MR venography. *J Magn Reson Imaging* 1998;8:630–633.
7. Monreal M, Alastrue A, Rull M, et al. Upper extremity deep venous thrombosis in cancer patients with venous access devices: prophylaxis with a low molecular weight heparin (Fragmin). *Thromb Haemost* 1996;75: 251–253.
8. Ferral H, Bjarnson H, Wholey M, et al. Recanalization of occluded veins to provide access for central catheter placement. *J Vasc Interv Radiol* 1996;7:681–685.
9. Funaki B, Zaleski GX, Leef JA, et al. Radiologic placement of long-term hemodialysis catheters in occluded jugular or subclavian veins or through patent thyrocervical collateral veins. *AJR* 1998;170:1194–1196.
10. Kaufman JA, Crenshaw WB, Kuter I, et al. Percutaneous placement of a central venous access device via an intercostal vein. *AJR* 1995;165:459–460.
11. Farrell T, Lang EV, Barnhart W. Sharp recanalization of central venous occlusions. *J Vasc Interv Radiol* 1999; 10:49–54.
12. Kenney PR, Dorfman GS, Denny DF Jr. Percutaneous inferior vena cava cannulation for long term parenteral access. *Surgery* 1985;97:602–605.
13. Denny DF Jr, Greenwood LH, Morse SS, et al. Inferior vena cava: translumbar catheterization for central venous access. *Radiology* 1989;170:1013–1014.
14. Lund GB, Lieberman RP, Haire WD, et al. Translumbar inferior vena cava catheters for long term venous access. *Radiology* 1990;174:31–35.
15. Bennett JD, Papadouris D, Rankin RN, et al. Percutaneous inferior vena caval approach for long-term cen-

tral venous access. *J Vasc Intervent Radiol* 1997;8: 851–855.

16. Rajan DK, Crouteau DL, Sturza SG, et al. Translumbar placement of inferior vena caval catheters: a solution for challenging hemodialysis access. *Radiographics* 1998;18:1155–1167.

17. Cazenave FL, Glass-Royal MC, Teitelbaum GP, et al. CT analysis of a safe approach for translumbar access to the aorta and inferior vena cava. *AJR* 1991;156: 395–396.

18. Crummy AB, Carlson P, McDermott JC, et al. Percutaneous transhepatic placement of a Hickman catheter [Letter]. *AJR* 1989;153:1317–1318.

19. Kaufman JA, Greenfield AJ, Fitzpatrick GF. Transhepatic cannulation of the inferior vena cava. *J Vasc Intervent Radiol* 1991;2:331–334.

20. Po CL, Koolpe HA, Allen S, et al. Transhepatic PermCath for hemodialysis. *Am J Kidney Dis* 1994;24:590–591.

21. Azizkhan RG, Taylor LA, Jaques PF, et al. Percutaneous translumbar and transhepatic inferior vena caval catheters for prolonged access in children. *J Pediatr Surg* 1992;27:165–169.

22. Bergey EA, Kaye RD, Reyes J, et al. Transhepatic insertion of vascular dialysis catheters in children: a safe, life-prolonging procedure. *Pediatr Radiol* 1999;29: 42–45.

23. Johnson JL, Fellows KE, Murphy JD. Transhepatic central venous access for cardiac catheterization and radiologic intervention. *Cathet Cardiovasc Diagn* 1995;35:168–171.

24. Pieters PC, Dittrich J, Prasad U, et al. Acute Budd-Chiari syndrome caused by percutaneous placement of a transhepatic inferior vena cava catheter. *J Vasc Intervent Radiol* 1997;8:587–590.

25. Friedman B, Kanter G, Titus D. Femoral venous catheters: a safe alternative for delivering parenteral nutrition. *Nutr Clin Pract* 1994;9:69–72.

26. Bertoglio S, Di Sommma C, Meszaros P, et al. Long-term femoral vein central venous access in cancer patients. *Eur J Surg Oncol* 1996;22:162–165.

27. Harden JL, Kemp L, Mirtallo J. Femoral catheters increase risk of infection in total parenteral nutrition patients. *Nutr Clin Pract* 1995;10:60–66.

28. Zaleski GX, Funaki B, Lorenz JM, et al. Experience with tunneled femoral hemodialysis catheters. *AJR* 1999;172:493–496.

29. Pippus KG, Giacomantonio JM, Gillis DA, et al. Thrombotic complications of saphenous central venous lines. *J Pediatr Surg* 1994;29:1218–1219.

30. Trottier SJ, Veremakis C, O'Brien J, et al. Femoral deep vein thrombosis associated with central venous catheterization: results from a prospective, randomized trial. *Crit Care Med* 1995;23:52–59.

31. Andrews JC. Percutaneous placement of a Hickman catheter with use of an intercostal vein for access. *J Vasc Intervent Radiol* 1994;5:859–861.

32. Meranze SG, McLean GK, Stein EJ, et al. Catheter placement in the azygous system: an unusual approach to venous access. *AJR* 1985;144:1075–1076.

33. Denny DF Jr. Central venous access via the hemiazygous vein. In: Trerotola SO, Savader SJ, Durham JD, eds. *Venous interventions.* Fairfax, VA: SCVIR, 1995: 507–510.

34. Racadio JM, Johnson ND, Doellman DA. Peripherally inserted central venous catheters: success of scalp-vein access in infants and newborns. *Radiology* 1999;210: 858–860.

35. Ikeda S, Sera Y, Oshiro H, et al. Transiliac catheterization of the inferior vena cava for long-term venous access in children. *Pediatr Surg Int* 1998;14:140–141.

36. Chang MY, Morris JB. Long-term central venous access through the ovarian vein. *J Parenter Enter Nutr* 1997;21:235–237.

37. Jaime-Solis E, Anaya-Ortega M, Moctezuma-Espinosa J. The internal mammary vein: an alternative route for central venous access with an implantable port. *J Pediatr Surg* 1994;29:1328–1330.

38. Malt RA, Kempster M. Direct azygous vein and superior vena cava cannulation for parenteral nutrition. *J Parenter Enter Nutr* 1983;7:580–581.

39. Oram-Smith JC, Mullen JL, Harken AH, et al. Direct right atrial catheterization for total parenteral nutrition. *Surgery* 1978;83:274–276.

40. Torosian MH, Meranze S, Mullen JL. Central venous access with occlusive central venous thrombosis. *Ann Surg* 1986;203:30–33.

Central Venous Access
Edited by Charles E. Ray, Jr.
Lippincott Williams & Wilkins, Philadelphia © 2001.

13

Central Venous Access: A Cost Analysis

*Charles E. Ray, Jr., MD and *†Jan Durham, MD

*Denver Health Medical Center;
*†University of Colorado Health Sciences Center, Denver, Colorado 80204

In the era of cost containment in health care, any new procedure that is performed must prove not only to be safe and efficacious, but must prove to be cost effective as well. In the not too distant past, radiologists perhaps more than most medical specialties benefited from the lack of active fiscal monitoring of new procedures. New technologies, such as many of the cross-sectional imaging modalities, were introduced into the medical marketplace without significant regard to the costs of such procedures. That era of medicine has likely passed, and the cost benefit of any new procedure or technology is becoming an ever increasingly more important variable. As Picus explained in a recent editorial, "No one pays for retail medical care today" (1).

DEFINITION OF TERMS

In order to discuss cost-related issues, definitions of commonly used terms must be presented. One must be careful when reading the medical literature; articles vary widely in not only their goals and conclusions, but also differ significantly in the methodology used.

The cost of a procedure can be separated into commonly used and reproducible components (Table 13.1). The monetary cost of any given procedure is the sum of three variables: variable direct cost, fixed direct cost, and fixed indirect cost (2). Variable direct cost represents those costs related to the performance of a procedure that may vary on a case-by-case basis, but are necessary for the performance of the procedure every time it is performed. An example of such costs would be the disposable tools used during a particular procedure. For example, although wires and sheaths are a necessary component of all tunneled catheter placements, using multiple wires rather than one wire would significantly increase the overall cost of the procedure. In a setting where time becomes an item that is charged (e.g., operating room or anesthesia charges), increasing the time necessary to complete the procedure would result in an increase in the variable direct costs as well. Fixed direct costs, by comparison, represent the overhead costs incurred by a hospital or other institution in order to be able and available to perform a procedure. An example of fixed direct costs would include wages for technical and nursing staff, equipment purchases, and maintenance contracts. Such costs are fixed because they are incurred whether or not the procedure is performed, but they may vary over time based on changes that occur within the infrastructure of an institution. For example, if the number of procedures decreases, the relative total fixed direct cost to an institution would increase per procedure if all other costs (e.g., number of technicians) remained constant. Finally, fixed indirect costs represent costs incurred by individual departments for maintenance of the physical plant in which the department resides (e.g. heating and cooling costs for the hospital). Fixed indirect costs do not change regardless of where a procedure is performed, unless concur-

TABLE 13.1. *Costs of medical procedures*

Cost				Charges
Nonmonetary costs	Monetary costs			
(e.g., discomfort, risk of complications, psychological factors)	Variable direct cost	Fixed direct cost	Fixed indirect cost	(what an institution bills for a procedure)
	(e.g., disposable tools)	(e.g., wages, maintenance)	(e.g., heating, lighting)	

rent changes are made to the physical plant, such as shutting off the power to an empty operating room. Fixed indirect costs therefore are generally unimportant when comparing surgically and radiologically placed central venous access devices (VADs).

It is vital when determining the cost of a procedure to be careful not to confuse cost with charges. Charges constitute what a hospital (or other billing body) expects to receive in return for services rendered. Charges may or may not be based on actual costs incurred for a procedure; typically, charges are higher than the cost for any given procedure. The reason for this disparity is an attempt by providing agencies such as hospitals to recoup the financial losses incurred by providing care to indigent patients or in the course of medical education. Charges may vary widely from one geographic region to another, and indeed may vary manifold between institutions within the same city.

One method by which hospital administrators may monitor procedures performed within their respective institutions is by evaluating relative value units (RVUs). RVUs represent an attempt to define and quantify the labor, time, and expertise required for the performance of certain procedures. Again, the problem with using RVUs to determine the cost of a procedure is that RVUs are typically used to determine the amount reimbursed to a hospital by Medicare rather than being representative of the cost incurred by a hospital or physician in performing the procedure.

The total cost of a procedure is even more difficult to determine than the complete monetary cost of a procedure. Included in the total cost of a procedure should be such nebulous variables as the benefits a patient derives from a procedure; the cost of any complications related to the procedure; the cost of care related to the procedure in its aftermath (e.g., long-term care for venous access devices); and the cost to the patient or institution for not undergoing the procedure. These nonmonetary costs are virtually impossible to quantify, and most investigators choose to ignore such variables. The cost of complications, as evidenced by the cost of treating the complication (e.g., antibiotics, thrombolytics) or the need to repeat a procedure, is likely the greatest cost related to this category. Interestingly, however, from the perspective of a patient, it is these nonmonetary variables that may determine the true value of any given procedure.

STREAMLINING COSTS

As discussed later, converting to radiologic placement of catheters that are placed in the operating room is one method by which to save considerable cost to the patient undergoing VAD placement. Other than an institution converting completely to radiologic placement of such devices, are there other methods by which to save costs on VAD placement procedures?

The utility of a routine postprocedure chest radiograph following VAD placement has recently come into question (3–5). In the past, particularly with a VAD placed either at the bedside or in the operating room without fluoroscopic guidance, a postprocedure chest radiograph was mandatory both to assess final catheter position as well as to determine whether or not a complication occurred during the procedure (e.g., pneumothorax, hemothorax). With the advent of radiologic placement of such devices using intermittent fluoroscopic guidance, as well as the increased use of the internal jugular vein approach, the value of obtaining a mandatory postprocedure chest radiograph has been questioned. In a study by Chang et al., 572 internal jugular catheter placements performed under sonographic and fluoroscopic guidance were retrospectively reviewed (4). In their series, a routine postprocedure chest radiograph demonstrated no complications (0%). A delayed second chest radiograph was obtained only if the patient became symptomatic; in this study, 2 (0.5%) patients demonstrated delayed pneumothoraces, neither of which were visible on the initial postprocedure chest radiograph.

In a more recent study by Lucey et al., 621 catheter placements under radiologic guidance were evaluated with routine postprocedure chest radiography (3). Included in this group were 63 catheters placed via a subclavian vein approach. In this study, 90 catheters demonstrated intraprocedural complications, such as sheath kinking, that were recognized and corrected during the initial catheter placement procedure. The only type of complication not noted during the actual catheter placement that was visualized on the postprocedure chest radiograph was catheter tip malposition (1% of placements). The total charges for the routine postprocedural chest radiographs in this series were over 15,000 Irish pounds.

Although routine chest radiographs are likely indicated following the initial placement of a VAD at the bedside, the necessity of obtaining a chest radiograph following line change over a wire has become controversial. A recent investigation from the surgical literature demonstrated only 3 of 1,301 (0.2%) catheter exchanges with an abnormality on the postprocedure chest radiograph; all three complications were catheter malpositions, but all three catheters were deemed useful in their initial position by the investigators (5).

Because a large percentage of the cost of surgically placed VADs is due to both variable and fixed direct costs (e.g., overhead), another method by which cost may be saved during catheter placement is by placing catheters outside of the normal surgical setting. Four studies from the surgical literature have attempted to change the way surgical lines are routinely placed as a method by which to decrease the cost of such procedures. In the first study, electrocardiography was used to guide placement of VADs (6). When compared with the control group (blind placement), a significant increase in ideal catheter tip location was achieved (96% vs. 59%; p < 0.001). Limitations to this study were the lack of fluoroscopic guidance in the control group, and the fact that 39% of the catheters placed in this study were catheter exchanges using an over-the-wire technique. A second study determined the cost savings of placing tunneled catheters at the bedside instead of placing them in the operating room (7). In this investigation, 55 Hickman catheters were placed in the operating room while 53 catheters were placed at the bedside. The complication rates were nearly identical, and savings of $1,545 in cost or charges were obtained per bedside placement. A separate similar study demonstrated a significant cost savings with arm ports placed at the bedside as compared with surgical placement in the operating room; in this study, there was no increase in the complication rate noted in the ports placed at the bedside (8). Finally, by simply streamlining the intraprocedural operating table setup (e.g., having a separate, smaller operating room supply pack with only the tools necessary for VAD placement), Howard et al. demonstrated a savings in supply costs of over $230 per patient (9).

RESULTS OF STUDIES COMPARING RADIOLOGIC VERSUS SURGICAL PLACEMENT OF VENOUS ACCESS DEVICES

Few studies have directly compared the two methods of catheter placement, and even fewer studies have been well-controlled and prospective by design. Again, care must be taken when reviewing the literature because many of the published studies compare hospital charges rather than the actual costs incurred during the procedure.

In a prelude to comparisons between radiologic and surgically placed lines, a study from

1984 compared VADs placed in the operating room using either the traditional cutdown technique or a completely percutaneous technique (10). Although a formal cost analysis was not performed, the authors demonstrated a greater than 50% decrease in operating time, an initial technical failure rate of only 4% in the percutaneous group, but 25% in the cutdown group, and no significant difference in complication rates. Although all of these catheters were placed in the operating room, this study demonstrated the efficacy of using a percutaneous approach.

Comparative studies between radiologic and surgical lines have been performed without formal cost analyses that demonstrate better success rates and lower complication rates with VADs placed under radiologic guidance than those placed surgically (11,12). In one of these studies, Nosher et al. demonstrated a slight decrease in hospital costs for radiologic placement as opposed to surgical lines ($1,531 vs. $1,826, respectively) (12). The methods of the cost analysis, as well as the statistical significance of the results, were not discussed in the article.

In a recent well-designed study, Noh et al. determined the true cost to the hospital of placement of tunneled hemodialysis catheters when placed both radiologically and surgically (13). In this study, the authors determined the direct (variable and fixed) and indirect costs for catheter placement. They demonstrated a total cost savings of $923 per patient; most of the savings ($569) came from the fixed indirect costs (e.g., reflecting the hospital overhead costs attributed to the individual department) (13). In a corollary to their first study and using the same strict cost-accounting methods, the same investigators demonstrated cost savings for chest port systems of $713 per port placed in the radiology department (2).

Although not comparing radiologic and surgically placed central VADs, an interesting study was performed to assess the cost effectiveness of peripherally inserted central catheters (PICCs) placed by interventional radiologists (14). In this study, the researchers assessed multiple strategies to determine at what cost level radiologic placement of PICCs becomes cost effective. Because many PICCs placed by nurses on the floor were either suboptimal or could not be used in their initial postprocedure position [53 of 150 (35%) in this study], it was determined that if the cost of the interventional radiology suite was less than $75, it was more cost effective to place all PICCs in the radiology department. In a letter to the editor directed toward the above study, Funaki and Zaleski pointed out that the long-term complications of using PICCs placed in a suboptimal position were not addressed (15); in the setting of increased complications with such suboptimal placements, it is likely that the level at which radiologic placement of PICCs becomes cost effective was underestimated.

Whether or not all PICCs, or indeed other VADs, should be placed under radiologic guidance remains open to debate. One factor that must be addressed is what type of procedure is not being performed in a room occupied by a patient undergoing a PICC placement. In other words, if a room is completely booked throughout the day and a department is unable to perform an angioplasty, for instance, because the room is occupied by PICC patients, then that particular PICC placement is not cost effective. If, however, a room is empty and fully staffed, the fixed direct and indirect costs have already been incurred by the hospital and it likely would be cost-effective to place the PICC even at a low level of compensation.

CONCLUSIONS

In the era of managed care and health cost containment, it is becoming increasingly important to evaluate the cost of radiologically performed procedures. Direct comparative studies are particularly helpful in convincing hospital administrators of the cost effectiveness of procedures performed in our departments. Although the true value of radiologic procedures ultimately depends on the safety and efficacy of such procedures, demonstration of their cost effectiveness can only help to convince administrators and third-party payers to support our efforts in patient care.

REFERENCES

1. Picus D. Comparing competing medical procedures: costs or charges—what should it matter? *Radiology* 1996;199:623–625.
2. Noh HM, Kaufman JA, Fan CM, et al. Radiological approach to central venous catheters: cost analysis. *Semin Intervent Radiol* 1998;15:335–340.
3. Lucey B, Varghese JC, Haslam P, et al. Routine chest radiographs after central line insertion: mandatory postprocedural evaluation or unnecessary waste of resources? *Cardiovasc Intervent Radiol* 1999;22:381–384.
4. Chang TC, Funaki B, Szymski GX. Are routine chest radiographs necessary after image-guided placement of internal jugular central venous access devices? *AJR* 1998;170:335–337.
5. Cullinane DC, Parkus DE, Reddy VS, et al. The futility of chest roentgenograms following routine central venous line changes. *Am J Surg* 1998;176:283–285.
6. Francis KR, Picard DL, Fajardo MA, et al. Avoiding complications and decreasing costs of central venous catheter placement utilizing electrocardiographic guidance. *Surg Gynecol Obstet* 1992;175:208–211.
7. Mannel RS, Manetta A, Hickman RL, et al. Cost analysis of Hickman catheter insertion at bedside in gynecologic oncology patients. *J Am Coll Surg* 1994;179:558–560.
8. Finney R, Albrink MH, Hart MB, et al. A cost-effective peripheral venous port system placed at the bedside. *J Surg Res* 1992;53:17–19.
9. Howard TJ, Stines CP, O'Connor JA, et al. Cost-effective supply use in permanent central venous catheter operations. *Am Surg* 1997;63:441–445.
10. Davis SJ, Thompson JS, Edney JA. Insertion of Hickman catheters. A comparison of cutdown and percutaneous techniques. *Am Surg* 1984;50:673–676.
11. McBride KD, Fisher R, Warnock N, et al. A comparative analysis of radiological and surgical placement of central venous catheters. *Cardiovasc Intervent Radiol* 1997;20:17–22.
12. Nosher JL, Shami MM, Siegel RL, et al. Tunneled central venous access catheter placement in the pediatric population: comparison of radiologic and surgical results. *Radiology* 1994;192:265–268.
13. Noh HM, Kaufman JA, Rhea JT, et al. Cost comparison of radiologic versus surgical placement of long-term hemodialysis catheters. *AJR* 1999;172:673–675.
14. Neuman ML, Murphy BD, Rosen MP. Bedside placement of peripherally inserted central catheters: a cost-effectiveness analysis. *Radiology* 1998:206:423–428.
15. Funaki B, Zaleski GX. Radiologic versus bedside placement of peripherally inserted central catheters. *Radiology* 1998:209:284–286.

Central Venous Access
Edited by Charles E. Ray, Jr.
Lippincott Williams & Wilkins, Philadelphia © 2001.

14

Complications of Central Venous Access Devices

Iftikhar Ahmad, MD and *Charles E. Ray, Jr., MD

Department of Radiology, Indiana University Medical Centre, Indianapolis, Indiana 46202;
°Denver Health Medical Center; University of Colorado Health Sciences Center, Denver, Colorado 80204

Central venous access devices have been in use since the early 1900s (1). With newer indications being added to a wide variety of uses for central venous catheters, these devices are being placed with a greater frequency. Today, over 3 million central venous catheters are placed each year in the United States alone, and an increasing numbers of these catheters are now placed in interventional radiology suits (2,3). Central venous access now constitutes a major portion of interventional radiology practice in many departments. Radiologists therefore have a duty to master the technique of central venous catheterization. They should be able to recognize and promptly treat the related complications.

A graphic presentation of complications of central venous access are depicted in Fig. 14.1.

PREOPERATIVE ASSESSMENT

Complications of central venous access can be minimized by detailed preoperative patient assessment. The operating physician should obtain a history of previous central venous catheter placements, including the site of catheter insertion and any subsequent complications. In particular, a history of venous thrombosis and catheter-related infection should be sought.

Patients with a history of previous central venous catheterization, particularly those with subsequent complications, should be screened using an imaging study such as duplex Doppler ultrasonography, contrast venography, or magnetic resonance venography. Documentation of patent central veins is imperative when placing tunneled dialysis catheters because of the high blood flow requirements. Patients with a history of central venous thrombosis, infection, previous trauma, or radiation therapy also should be investigated for vascular patency.

A directed physical examination should be performed to include assessment of the neck and upper extremities for evidence of central venous thrombosis or infection. The signs of central venous occlusion include edema of the upper extremities, pain or discomfort in the affected limb, and dilatation of superficial venous collateral vessels.

Infection should be suspected if there are signs of induration, erythema, or frank pus. In the case of entry site or tunnel infection of a previous catheter, it is preferable to choose a healthy skin puncture site. If the patient has catheter-induced septicemia, a tunneled catheter or totally implanted venous access device should not be placed until the infection has been treated. Instead, a temporary nontunneled catheter may be placed until such time that the systemic infection is completely resolved.

Absolute neutropenia (<1,000/mL) and thrombocytopenia (<50,000/mL) are considered contraindications for tunneled and totally implanted venous access placement. We prefer an international normalized ratio (INR) of less

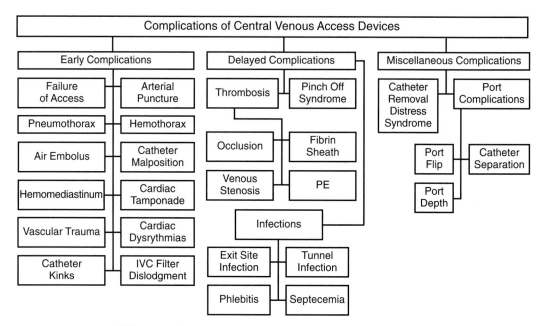

FIG. 14.1. Complications of central venous access devices.

than 1.3 for elective tunneled catheters; temporary nontunneled catheters can safely be placed with a platelet count of less than 50,000/mL and higher INR values, especially via the internal jugular vein (4).

Additional details concerning preprocedure patient evaluation are discussed elsewhere in this book (Chapter 3).

EARLY CATHETER INSERTION-RELATED COMPLICATIONS

Because some of the early complications related to catheter insertion can be potentially fatal, their prompt recognition and treatment is imperative. Early complications include failure to gain access, pneumothorax, arterial puncture, air embolus, catheter tip malposition, cardiac dysrhythmias, mediastinal, pleural and pericardial hemorrhage, dislodgment of an inferior vena cava filter, and catheter/peel-away sheath kinks.

Failure to Gain Access

In nonradiologic settings, central venous catheters are placed using external anatomic landmarks (5). Failure to gain venous access in these settings is encountered in up to 13% of cases; the number of unsuccessful attempts increases significantly when catheters are placed in emergency situations (6). Ultrasonography or venograpic guidance used in radiology departments to gain vascular access has decreased the number of unsuccessful attempts. According to one study, more than two attempts at venous puncture were required in 7.3% cases when ultrasonographic guidance was used, compared with 24.8% of cases when anatomic landmarks were used (7). The rate of complications increases from 4.3% with one needle pass to 24% with two or more needle passes (7).

An attempt at venous puncture without imaging guidance may fail because of improper technique, variant anatomy, or deformity of the external anatomic landmarks, such as may be seen following fracture of the clavicle (8). In about 5.5% cases, the internal jugular vein does not lie in the path predicted by anatomic landmarks (9).

In addition to guiding venous access, ultrasonography or venography also confirms the patency of the vessel being accessed prior to attempting venous puncture. Occlusion of the vein being accessed should be suspected when there is a history of previous central catheterizations, radiation, or surgery. Occlusion of the central veins may not always be symptomatic.

In the event of thrombosis of central veins, alternative routes of venous access are used. Transfemoral, translumbar, and transhepatic routes, as well as dilated collateral veins, can be used once the subclavian and internal jugular routes have been exhausted (10). More complicated venous access can be achieved by placing catheters via intercostal veins into the azygous or hemiazygous veins. Aggressive surgical approaches may include direct catheter placement into the right atrium (11).

Alternatively, recanalization of the occluded vein may be attempted using either a guidewire-catheter combination (12), or by sharp recanalization of the occluded central vein (13).

Pneumothorax

Pneumothorax accounts for 30% of all complications encountered with non-imaging-guided central venous puncture, and is more likely to occur with blind subclavian venous puncture than internal jugular venous access (14). Up to 6% of patients undergoing non-imaging-guided central catheter placement develop a pneumothorax; however, by using imaging guidance, the rate of pneumothorax can be reduced to 1.6% or less (15). Pneumothorax should especially be suspected if air is aspirated while attempting to access the subclavian vein.

Most pneumothorices caused during central venous catheter placement remain asymptomatic. A pneumothorax may not be demonstrable on an immediate postprocedure radiograph; in some patients, pneumothorax may not be visible up to 6 days postprocedure (8). Central venous catheter placement may be followed by an immediate postprocedure chest radiograph; if this radiograph demonstrates a pneumothorax of less than 30%, conservative management is generally indicated. Patients are observed for 4 hours, followed by discharge if the follow-up radiograph does not demonstrate any increase

in the size of the pneumothorax, and there is no change in symptomatology. If, however, the initial pneumothorax is larger than 30%, there is an increase in the size of pneumothorax on the delayed 4-hour chest radiography, or if the patient is symptomatic, a chest tube should be placed (16).

In our practice, a 7 French (Fr) multihole pigtail catheter is placed into the pleural cavity. The catheter is then attached to a Heimlich valve (Cook, Inc., Bloomington, IN, U.S.A.). We prefer to aspirate all the air from the pleural cavity and leave the Heimlich valve in place. A follow-up radiograph is obtained at 4 hours, followed by radiographs every 12 hours. After the pneumothorax has resolved, the Heimlich valve is removed and the chest tube is capped. A repeat chest radiograph is obtained after 4 hours; if the follow-up radiograph remains negative, the chest tube is removed.

Arterial Puncture

Inadvertent arterial puncture is the second most common complication of non-imaging-guided central venous access (14). The reported incidence of arterial punctures performed without imaging guidance can be as high as 7% (15). It may not always be possible to recognize pulsatile blood return from an arterial puncture, particularly if a 21-gauge micropuncture needle is used.

In most cases, arterial injury following needle puncture heals spontaneously. However, in some instances serious and potentially fatal complications may occur. Injury to the arterial wall following needle puncture can lead to pseudoaneurysm or arteriovenous fistula formation. In more severe cases, hemothorax, mediastinal hematoma, or extrapleural hematoma may result (17–19). Occasionally, trauma to the carotid artery can cause dissection and thrombosis of the vessel leading to stroke (20). Death due to arterial injury during central venous catheter placement has been reported (21).

Air Embolus

Large volumes of air can enter the central veins during catheter insertion or exchange. Air embolism is most likely to occur when large peel-away sheaths are used for central venous catheter placement. Meticulous attention to technique (e.g., placing the patient in the Trendelenburg position and having the patient perform a Valsalva maneuver during catheter insertion) minimizes the chance of air embolus (22). It is important at all times to keep the needle, dilator, or sheath occluded, either with a wire or gloved finger. The chances of air embolus are greatest while attempting to insert the catheter through the peel-away sheath after having withdrawn the guidewire and the stiffener. Pinching the sheath halfway down the exposed shaft while removing the stiffener and guidewire, and keeping the sheath pinched until the catheter has been inserted, minimizes the chance of air embolus. It is also important to remember to clamp each limb of the catheter following the initial preparatory flush.

The chance of air embolus increases in patients with low central venous pressure. For instance, 14 Fr catheters can aspirate air at the rate of 100 cc/s with a pressure gradient of only 5 cm of water (23). The minimum amount of air that can cause fatal air embolism is uncertain, but death has been reported with as little as 100 cc of air (24).

Patients developing air embolus immediately start coughing and develop respiratory distress; if severe, they rapidly become hemodynamically unstable. These patients should be immediately placed in the left lateral decubitus position to trap the air in the right atrium. Putting the patient in the Trendelenburg position also helps prevent air crossing the tricuspid valve into the right ventricle. A large-bore central venous catheter has been used to acutely aspirate as much air as possible from the right atrium (25).

Catheter Tip Malposition

Regardless of the site of entry, the tip of the central venous catheters should ideally be placed at the superior vena cava (SVC)-right atrial junction. Placement of the catheter tip in the subclavian vein is associated with a higher rate of venous thrombosis. A catheter placed

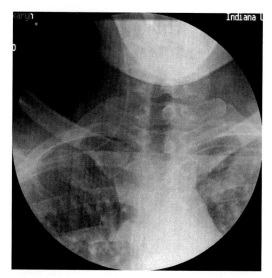

FIG. 14.2. Peripherally inserted central catheter placed without fluoroscopic guidance at the bedside with the tip in the ipsilateral internal jugular vein.

too far into the right atrium can cause endocardial trauma, leading to valvular damage and sterile or septic vegetations (26,27). Catheters placed with the tip in the heart can also lead to cardiac dysrhythmias and even cardiac perforation.

Catheter tip malposition may occur at the time of insertion if the catheter placement is performed without fluoroscopic guidance, or later due to movement of soft tissues of the patient's chest wall, changes in posture, or respiratory movements (14). Catheter placement without fluoroscopic guidance has been shown to lead to malposition of the tip in up to 32% of cases (28).

Malposition of the central venous catheter tip is most common with peripherally inserted central catheters (PICCs). The catheter tip may be placed in a small tributary of the subclavian vein, the ipsilateral internal jugular vein (Fig. 14.2), or the contralateral subclavian vein (29,30). PICCs are more likely to be malpositioned because they are more commonly placed at the bedside without fluoroscopic guidance, and because the catheters are smaller, softer, more flexible, and have a longer intravascular course. Larger bore tunneled or nontunneled catheters placed into central veins are less likely to be positioned in a small tributary or in the contralateral internal jugular vein.

Vascular Perforation, Hemomediastinum, Hemothorax, and Cardiac Tamponade

Vascular perforation during catheter placement, or subsequently due to erosion by the catheter tip, can lead to mediastinal hematoma or cardiac tamponade (31,32). Intrathoracic bleeding in the form of hemomediastinum, hemothorax, or hemopericardium can be fatal if unrecognized.

Hemomediastinum occurs in less than 1% of central venous catheter insertions (4). The vascular injury is generally self-contained because of a tamponading effect of the mediastinal hematoma. Postprocedure chest radiography demonstrates a widened mediastinum. Free blood return before starting to use the catheter confirms the intravascular location of the catheter.

Vascular injury during catheter insertion is most likely to occur with the stiff introducer sheaths, which may not follow the course of the guidewire. Using a stiff guidewire with a straight tip also may cause vascular injury. Stiffer and less biocompatible catheter materials, such as polyurethane, may cause delayed vascular erosion. Due to greater catheter stiffness, larger bore catheters increase the risk of vascular trauma (33). Movement of the catheter tip in the superior vena cava with change in posture also may contribute to vascular trauma (34).

Cardiac Dysrhythmias

Manipulating the guidewire or catheter while in contact with the endocardium of the right atrium or ventricle may induce a cardiac dysrhythmia during central venous catheter placement. A significant number of patients experience atrial (41%) or ventricular (25%) dysrhythmias when central venous catheters are placed without imaging guidance (35). Dysrhythmias encountered in such settings are usually transient and asymptomatic, but the nurse or assistant present during the procedure should keep a vigilant eye on the monitor to detect dysrhythmias. As soon as any irregularity is noted, the guidewire or the catheter should be promptly withdrawn from the heart. Persistent dysrhythmias should be promptly treated using standard Advanced Cardiac Life Support (ACLS) protocol.

Catheter and Peel-Away Sheath Kinks

The peel-away sheaths are designed to have a large inner lumen and relatively thin walls made of stiff material. Although these properties facilitate catheter insertion, they make the sheaths prone to kink. A kink in the peel-away sheath occurs when the inner stiffener has been removed prior to catheter placement. A kink in the peel-away sheath precludes advancement of the catheter, and may occur at the vascular access site or, in the case of subclavian venous puncture, may occur at the junction of the subclavian and internal jugular veins. The right internal jugular vein offers a straight approach to the heart. Catheters placed through the right internal jugular vein do not have to negotiate any acute angles and therefore infrequently encounter the kinking problem.

If a kink in the peel-away introducer sheath is encountered, one should attempt to pass a hydrophilic guidewire through the catheter and across the kink to add to the stiffness of the catheter. By doing so, the catheter–guidewire combination may have enough stiffness to straighten the kink. Alternatively, the sheath may be withdrawn until the kink lies in a relatively straight portion of the vessel or in an extravascular location while maintaining vascular access by the distal portion of the sheath. This maneuver also typically straightens the kink. A safety guidewire should be placed to secure vascular access in case the peel-away sheath is withdrawn completely outside the vessel.

After the catheter is placed and the sheath removed, a kink in the catheter itself can occur if the catheter makes an acute turn. For tunneled catheters, the acute curve in the path may occur at the site of venous entry. Subclavian catheters make a gentler curve and are less likely to kink; internal jugular catheters on the other hand make a more acute turn and are liable to kink. The curvature of the catheter as it gently arches

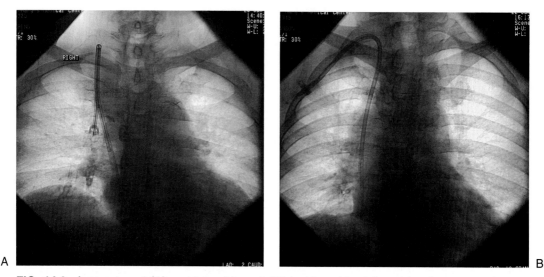

FIG. 14.3. A parasternal **(A)** and lateral tunnel **(B)** fashioned for internal jugular access demonstrate a smooth curvature of the catheter without any kink.

over the clavicle generally prevents a kink. (Fig. 14.3).

Vena Cava Filter Dislodgment

Inferior vena cava, and more recently superior vena cava, filters may become dislodged during central venous catheter placement (36). When the central venous catheters are placed without fluoroscopic guidance, the potential of dislodging previous placed vena cava filters always exists. This complication is especially common when using a J-curve guidewire, because the curved wire tip can be entrapped within the struts of an inferior vena cava filter. Physicians placing central venous catheters may not be aware of the presence of a vena cava filter. Therefore, if any resistance is encountered during catheter placement, it is imperative for the physician to visualize the guidewire and catheter tip under fluoroscopy to evaluate the cause of the resistance. According to one study, stainless-steel Greenfield filters and Vena Tech filters are at a greater risk for dislodgment (37).

DELAYED COMPLICATIONS

Twenty percent to 35% of tunneled catheters are removed prior to completion of therapy due to delayed complications (38). Delayed complications include thrombotic complications, infectious complications, catheter fracture, and catheter impingement syndrome. Thrombotic complications can be further divided into catheter occlusion, fibrin sheath, venous thrombosis, venous stenosis, and pulmonary embolism. Infectious complications can be further divided into exit site infection, tunnel infection, infectious thrombophlebitis, and septicemia.

Thrombotic Complications

Multiple factors contribute to thrombosis and subsequent stenosis or occlusion of the central veins. Contributing factors for catheter-induced thrombosis include route of venous access, biocompatibility of the catheter material, size and length of the catheter, and the length of time the catheter stays in place (39). Other factors promoting venous thrombosis include a hypercoagulable state that may be secondary to the underlying condition for which the catheter was placed, hypovolemia, venous stasis, infection, and frequency and the type of medications infused through the catheter (40).

The incidence of central venous stenosis ranges from 3% to 15% with internal jugular catheters to 15% to 40% with catheters inserted via the subclavian vein (41). The most likely cause for this discrepancy is perpetual microtrauma caused by the catheter at the insertion site secondary to chest wall movement by respiration or arm movement. Internal jugular catheters are less likely to move with chest wall motion and thus are less likely to cause central venous stenosis.

Biocompatibility of the catheter material may alter the thrombogenecity of the catheter. Catheters made of polyurethane and polyethylene are less biocompatible and theoretically may lead to a higher incidence of venous stenosis. Silicone is softer and has greater biocompatibility; it is therefore used in the manufacture of tunneled catheters for long-term use.

Fibrin Sheath

The human body recognizes intravascular catheters as a foreign body, and responds by enveloping the catheter within a fibrin sheath. Virtually all central venous catheters develop a fibrin sheath covering the shaft of the catheter to some extent. The fibrin sheath generally extends from the site of venous puncture to the tip of the catheter. It becomes symptomatic if it overhangs the tip of the catheter, thereby forming a flap that functions as a one-way valve. The catheter can be flushed using positive pressure, but negative pressure generated to aspirate blood displaces the fibrin sheath over the catheter tip and effectively occludes the catheter. In this manner the diagnosis of a fibrin sheath can be made clinically. Radiologic confirmation involves infusing contrast slowly through the catheter while imaging over the catheter tip. In the presence of a fibrin sheath, contrast is seen tracking back along the shaft of the catheter instead of exiting from the tip. (Fig. 14.4). If a contrast injection is made while removing the catheter, the entire sheath can occasionally be visualized after catheter removal. The significance of this residual intravascular fibrin sheath after catheter removal is uncertain. Catheter exchanges may be compromised by placing the new catheter into the previous fibrin sheath if an over-the-wire catheter exchange technique is used. In some instances, mechanical disruption

of the fibrin sheath prior to placement of the new catheter may be advantageous.

At our institutions, fibrin sheaths are initially treated with tissue plasminogen activator (TPA). One milligram of TPA diluted in 1–2 mL of saline is injected into each catheter lumen. The TPA is allowed to dwell for 1 hour before aspiration is attempted. Patients in whom this initial TPA therapy is unsuccessful undergo a TPA infusion. To perform infusion therapy, 5 mg of TPA is diluted in 100 mL of saline, which is infused at a rate of 20 mL/h through each lumen for 2½ hours. The total TPA dose is therefore 5 mg for a double-lumen catheter.

If TPA therapy is unsuccessful, the fibrin sheath can be mechanically disrupted either with a balloon or by stripping the sheath. Balloon disruption of the sheath is performed when the existing catheter is being exchanged over a wire for a new catheter. A stiff hydrophilic wire is placed through each lumen of the existing catheter. The existing catheter is removed, and a balloon catheter is inserted over each wire. The ball catheter may possess either a compliant or a noncompliant balloon. The balloon is inflated and the catheter is moved back and forth in order to disrupt the sheath. The same maneuver is repeated for the second wire. An additional method by which to mechanically disrupt the fibrin sheath is by catheter stripping. Using a femoral vein approach, a gooseneck snare is advanced into the superior vena cava. The tip of the catheter is encircled, and the snare is advanced along the shaft of the catheter as far proximally as possible. The snare is then closed and withdrawn in order to cut through the fibrin sheath. Care must be taken not to grasp the catheter too tightly, or the snare may actually fracture the catheter. The procedure is repeated multiple times in order to debulk as much of the fibrin sheath as possible.

Catheter Occlusion

Central venous catheters are usually flushed with a heparin solution so that the entire catheter lumen is occupied with the anticoagulant. If, however, blood refluxes into the catheter lumen, it can clot and occlude the catheter

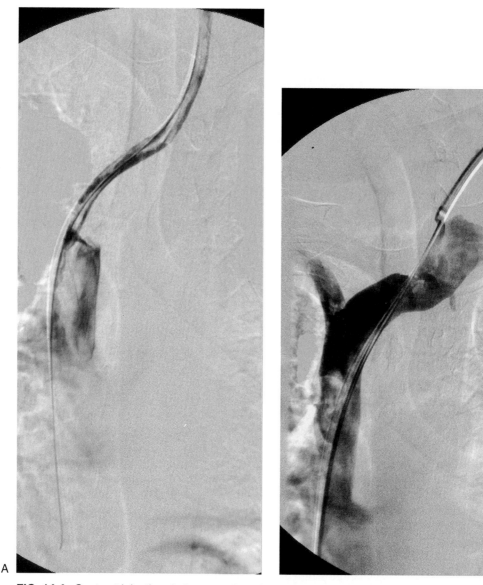

A   B

FIG. 14.4. Contrast injection during over-the-wire exchange of a tunneled dialysis catheter in a 38-year-old male demonstrates a long fibrin sheath extending from the venotomy site to the right atrium. Contrast was injected after pulling the catheter in to the innominate vein over a safety wire (**A**). Fibrin sheath was disrupted using an over-the-wire Fogarty balloon. After exchanging the catheter over the wire, contrast injection was again performed which demonstrates complete disruption of the fibrin sheath (**B**).

lumen. Therefore, it is important to lock the catheter while still infusing heparin solution so that blood does not reflux back into the lumen. This is done by keeping positive pressure on the infusion syringe plunger until the syringe is removed from the catheter hub.

Catheter occlusions can be treated by using thrombolytic therapy. TPA diluted to 1 mg/mL is injected into each lumen to fill the lumen. The TPA is allowed to dwell for 1 hour before the catheter is checked for patency. In addition, the catheter should be flushed with a 1-mL tuberculin syringe with a leur-lock connection, because a 1-mL syringe can generate up to 22 atmospheres of pressure and may be able to dislodge the clot. If the TPA dwell does not clear the thrombus, a TPA infusion as outlined above may be performed.

Central Venous Thrombosis and Occlusion

Catheter-induced central venous thrombosis is a major cause of chronic venous occlusions. The factors contributing to thrombosis and occlusion of the central veins include endothelial trauma caused by venous puncture and subsequent dilatation of the tract for catheter insertion (42); biocompatibility of the catheter material (39); duration of catheterization (39); and, in the case of the subclavian vein, the torque of the catheter over the first rib and to-and-fro movement of the catheter with each cardiac contraction and respiratory movement (41).

Venous stenosis or occlusion secondary to central venous catheters is more common with catheter insertion into the subclavian vein than into the internal jugular vein (Fig. 14.5) (41). Up to 53% of subclavian venous catheters may be associated with central venous stenosis or occlusion (43), but only a small percentage of these patients become clinically symptomatic. Up to 5% of patients may present with arm swelling and prominent collateral veins under the skin (44). In most instances, these clinical symptoms subside without further intervention, and in the absence of clinical symptoms, central venous stenosis is rarely diagnosed, much less treated. Exceptions to this conservative approach are patients in chronic renal failure who may require an arteriovenous (AV) fistula or graft in the ipsilateral arm. Symptomatic patients may require anticoagulation or catheter-directed thrombolytic therapy; resistant cases may be treated with venous angioplasty and or stent placement (45, 46). Occluded central veins can occasionally be traversed with a guidewire-catheter combination. Once the occluded venous segment has been negotiated, the vein may be primarily stented with a flexible self-expanding stent. Resilient stenotic segments have

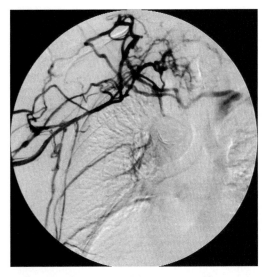

FIG. 14.5. A 38-year-old asymptomatic woman with a history of multiple central venous catheters for chemotherapy infusion because of malignant melanoma. An upper extremity venogram was performed after an unsuccessful attempt at subclavian Hickman catheter placement. Multiple collateral vessels are visualized draining into the contralateral internal jugular vein.

been recanalized with sharp needle and guidewire combinations with some success (13).

In our practice, patients with central venous occlusion are treated conservatively for 48 to 72 hours. Unless contraindicated, most patients are given low-molecular-weight heparin (30–60 mg twice daily). Waiting for 48 to 72 hours allows collateral veins to develop in the majority of patients and their clinical signs and symptoms to resolve. In patients who are resistant to this initial form of therapy, catheter-directed thrombolysis or catheter removal might be necessary.

Pulmonary Embolism

Deep venous thrombosis of the lower extremity accounts for the majority of pulmonary emboli (PEs), most likely because of greater incidence of thrombosis of the lower extremity. However, because of increasing use of central venous catheters, thrombosis of the deep veins of the upper extremity is becoming more common (47). Although the risk for such emboli causing clinically significant PEs remains debatable, one investigator concluded that 36% of patients with upper extremity deep venous thrombosis demonstrate evidence of PEs (48). Most of the PEs in this study were clinically silent.

INFECTIOUS COMPLICATIONS

Infection of central venous access devices is the most frequently encountered delayed complication (49). Infectious complications are thought to be related to the initial procedure when they occur within 2 weeks of catheter placement. Infections after 2 weeks are attributed to nonsterile technique during subsequent catheter use. Infectious complications can be divided into exit site infection, referring to infections within 2 cm of the exit site; tunnel infections, occurring beyond 2 cm from the exit site; infectious thrombophlebitis and; catheter-induced septicemia.

Exit site infections and tunnel infections may present as erythema or frank abscess around the catheter exit site. Septic thrombophlebitis presents as inflamed and indurated linear markings overlying the inflamed vein. The diagnosis of catheter-related systemic infection might not be straightforward. Indirect evidence of catheter infection can be obtained by cultures from the blood drawn from the catheter and from peripheral blood. The culture specimen obtained from the catheter yields 10 times as many colonies as grown from the peripheral blood sample. A firm diagnosis of catheter-induced septicema involves catheter removal and catheter tip culture.

Exit site infections occur in up to 45% of patients and are usually treated with oral antibiotics; tunnel infections occur in up to 20% of patients, and catheter-induced septicema can be seen in up to 50% of cases (50). Tunnel infections and catheter-induced septicema are generally given an initial trial of intravenous antibiotic therapy; in most cases, however, adequate treatment of tunnel infections and septicemia requires catheter removal. Septic thrombophlebitis is a rare complication occurring in up to 3.5% of cases and may be treated with a trial of warm compresses, antiinflammatory medications, and antibiotics. Once septic thrombophlebitis is diagnosed, therapy consists of catheter removal and a long (e.g., 6 weeks) course of intravenous antibiotic therapy.

The incidence of procedure-related catheter infections is comparable among catheters placed in the radiology and operating suites (50). For obvious reasons, catheter-related infections occur more frequently in patients who are immunosuppressed and in patients with a white blood cell count of less than 2,000/mL or greater than 20,000/mL (51). Catheters with multiple lumens are associated with higher rates of infection, possibly due to greater handling of such catheters and the underlying condition requiring multilumen catheters in the first place (52). The route chosen for venous access also plays an important role in the incidence of catheter-related infections. Subclavian catheters are least likely to get infected, where the rate of catheter colonization is 10%. Higher infection rates are noted with internal jugular (22%) and femoral vein (47%) access (40). Use of semipermeable transparent dressing also may increase the risk of infection by producing warm moist conditions suitable for bacterial growth.

Use of prophylactic antibiotics and silver-impregnated collagen cuff in tunneled catheters has significantly reduced the incidence of catheter-related infections (53).

Pinch-Off Syndrome Catheter Fragmentation and Catheter Embolization

Catheter fragmentation is rare. The factors leading to catheter fracture include biocompatibility of the catheter material, degradation of the catheter with time, and mechanical factors such as pinch-off syndrome. Medications injected through the catheter, particularly chemotherapeutic agents, also may degrade the catheter material. Long-term central venous catheters fracture at a site of stress, which is usually at the site of entry into the vein or an acute bend in the catheter. The introduction of softer and more biocompatible silicone catheters has re-

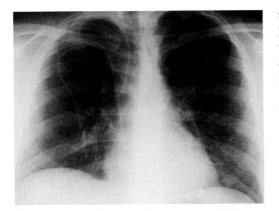

FIG. 14.6. Chest radiograph of a 41-year-old man with a history of malignant malinoma. A chest radiograph was obtained because of difficulty in withdrawing blood from the chest port. The chest radiograph shows grade 2 pinch-off of the subclavian catheter. A chest radiograph obtained a week earlier (not shown) did not demonstrate any abnormality. A follow-up chest radiograph obtained 2 days later showed the catheter fragmented and embolized to the pulmonary artery.

duced the incidence of catheter degradation and fragmentation.

Pinch-off syndrome occurs in catheters placed through a subclavian vein when the site of venous entry is medial. As the name suggests, the catheter is pinched between the first rib and the clavicle (Fig. 14.6). If the catheter enters the vein lateral to the first rib, it is protected by blood in the subclavian vein, and catheter pinch-off will not occur. If, however, the entry site is more medial, the catheter is unprotected as it enters the clavicular–first rib space. The severity of catheter impingement can be graded from grade 0, indicating no radiographically visible deformity of the catheter, to grade 3, indicating complete transection of the catheter (54).

Catheter fracture is usually asymptomatic. The fractured fragment is often identified incidentally on a routine chest radiograph. Catheter fracture is sometimes recognized for the first time when the entire catheter is not retrieved from the body at the time of removal.

Interventional radiologists have spent many hours trying to retrieve fractured catheters from the pulmonary artery. If the catheter fracture is known to be recent, an attempt should be made to retrieve the catheter to prevent perforation/erosion of the pulmonary artery. A catheter fragment lodged in the pulmonary artery can act as a nidus for infection or future thromboembolic events. If, however, the catheter has been in the pulmonary artery for a long time, it becomes covered with endothelium and may be impossible to retrieve.

Catheter retrieval is usually performed using a gooseneck snare. Retrieval is relatively easy if one end of the catheter fragment is free from the vessel wall so that the snare can encircle the catheter. If both ends of the catheter are flush against the vessel wall, however, catheter retrieval becomes quite tedious. Curved catheters can be used in an attempt to dislodge one end of the fractured fragment. A guidewire can be passed through the curved catheter around the middle of the shaft of the fractured fragment; the guidewire is then ensnared, effectively capturing the fractured catheter from the middle of the shaft (Fig. 14.7).

MISCELLANEOUS COMPLICATIONS

Miscellaneous complications include complications specific to totally implanted ports, and a set of complications classified as central venous catheter removal distress syndrome.

Complications Specific to Totally Implanted Ports

Totally implanted ports are now frequently being placed in radiology suites using imaging guidance. Implanted ports can be placed in the arm or the chest. These devices carry the risk of the same early and delayed group of complications as encountered with other venous access devices, but there is an additional set of complications limited only to the totally implanted ports. These complications include flipping of the port reservoir, separation of the port reservoir from the catheter, too deep or superficial reservoir placement, and skin dehiscence over the reservoir (40).

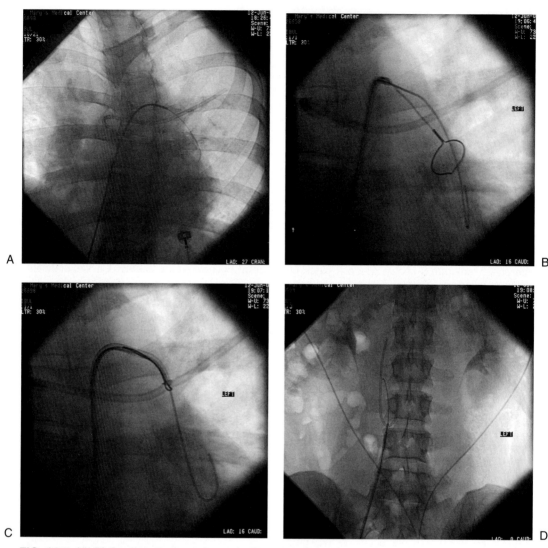

FIG. 14.7. (A–D) Same patient as shown in Fig. 14.6. Pulmonary artery foreign body retrieval was performed using a gooseneck snare. (Images courtesy of Dr. Bob Vogt, M.D.)

Totally implanted ports are composed of a reservoir and a catheter. The reservoir has a flat metallic or plastic surface resting on the chest wall or against a hard surface in the arm (e.g., the biceps fascia). The opposite convex surface is formed by a thick silicone diaphragm, which is punctured by a non-coring needle to gain access. Once the ports are placed and the skin closed over the reservoir, there is a small risk that the reservoir would invert, making puncture of the silicone diaphragm impossible. The

port reservoir is most likely to flip if the subcutaneous pocket is too generous. Almost all port manufacturers provide holes on the port reservoir to place stay sutures if the operator so desires. However, we do not place stay sutures; instead, we prefer to initially fashion the pocket smaller than the port, and enlarge the subcutaneous pocket by blunt dissection using the port reservoir itself. Therefore, the port sits snugly in the pocket and does not flip. If stay sutures are placed, as some operators prefer, they may be very difficult to find and remove at the time of port removal.

Unlike most other venous access devices, the port reservoir and the catheter may be provided in the kit as separate items and have to be assembled at the time of implantation. The catheter is attached to the reservoir using a locking mechanism. If improperly applied, or in the setting of failure of the locking mechanism, the connection between the catheter and the port reservoir may become loose and the injected material may spill into the subcutaneous port pocket.

When implanting the port, the depth at which the port reservoir is placed has to be fashioned so that the port is easily palpable through the skin and the Huber needle is able to reach the reservoir without difficulty. If on the other hand, the reservoir is placed too superficially, the skin over the reservoir may break down, exposing the port. If placed too deeply, the port may be impossible to palpate and inaccessible to the Huber needle.

Central Venous Device Removal Complications

A rare but potentially fatal set of complications has been described as central venous catheter removal distress syndrome. In this syndrome, removal of a central venous catheter may be associated with neurocardiopulmonary distress. Kim et al. described seven patients who developed central venous catheter removal distress syndrome (55). The complications included neurologic paresis or coma, respiratory failure, and shock. The complications occurred following complete removal of the catheter, or after introduction of the guidewire for catheter removal. A mortality rate of 12.5% has been reported for central venous catheter removal distress syndrome.

The etiology of central venous catheter removal distress syndrome is presumed to be air embolism. Central venous catheter removal, just like catheter insertion, requires meticulous care to prevent air embolism. The patient should be asked to perform the Valsalva maneuver during catheter removal and the skin entry site should be sealed with Xeroform petrolatum dressing (Sherwood Medical St. Louis, MO). The incidence of this syndrome is unknown but is likely exceedingly rare.

REFERENCES

1. Kalso E. A short history of central venous catheterization. *Acta Anaesth Scand* 1985;81(suppl):7–10.
2. Scott WL Complications associated with central venous catheters: a survey. *Chest* 1988;94:1221–1224.
3. Lund GB, Trerotola SO, Scheel PF, et. al. Outcome of tunneled hemodialysis catheters placed by radiologists. *Radiology* 1996;198:467–472.
4. Mansfield PF, Hohn DC, Fornage BD, et al. Complications and failures of subclavian-vein catheterization. *N Engl J Med* 1994;331:1735–1738.
5. Nelson EW. Venous access techniques. *Urol Clin North Am* 1986;13:475–487.
6. Bo-Lin GW, Anderson DJ, Anderson KC, et al. Percutaneous central venous catheterization performed by medical house officers: a prospective study. *Cathet Cardiovasc Diagn* 1982;8:23–29.
7. Denys BG, Uretsky BF, Reddy Ps. Ultrasound-assisted cannulation of the internal jugular vein: a prospective comparison to the external landmark-guided technique. *Circulation* 1993;87:1557–1562.
8. Whiteman ED. Complications associated with use of central venous access devices. *Curr Probl Surg* 1996;33:319–378.
9. Denys BG, Uretsky BF. Anatomical variations of internal jugular vein location: impact on central venous access. *Crit Care Med* 1991;19:1516–1519.
10. Patel NH. Alternative approaches to central venous access. *Semin Intervent Radiol* 1998;15:325–333.
11. Groman RC, Buzby GP. Difficult access problems. *Surg Oncol Clin North Am* 1995;4:453–472.
12. Vedantham S. Endovascular strategies for superior vena cava obstruction. *Tech Vasc Intervent Radiol* 2000;3:29–39.
13. Lang EV, Farrel T, Vrachliotis TG, et al. Sharp recanalization for chronic central venous occlusions. *Tech Vasc Intervent Radiol* 2000;3:21–28.
14. Mitchell SE, Clark RA. Complications of central venous catheters. *AJR* 1979:133:467–476.
15. Bjarnason H, Lehmann S. Central venous access. In: Castaneda-Zuniga WR, Tadavarthy SM, eds. *Interventional radiology.* Baltimore: Williams & Wilkins, 1992: 941–961.
16. Morton JE, Jan-Mohammed RMI, Barker HE, et al. Percutaneous insertion of subclavian Hickman catheters. *Bone Marrow Transplant* 1991;7:39–41.
17. Owens CA, Yaghmai B, Warner D. Complications of central venous catheterization. *Semin Intervent Radiol* 1998;15:341–355.
18. Yerdel MA, Karayalcin K, Aras N, et al. Mechanical complications of subclavian vein catheterization. A prospective study. *Int Surg* 1991;76:18–22.
19. Lacqua MJ, Sahdev P. Widened mediastinum in acute trauma: a complication of subclavian vein catheterization. *J Emerg Med* 1994;12:607–609.
20. Hurwitz BJ, Posner JB, Cerebral infarction complicating subclavian vein catheterization. *Ann Neurol* 1977;1:253–264.

21. Pessa ME, Howard RJ. Complication of Hickman-Broviac catheters. *Surg Gynecol Obstet* 1985;161:257–260.

22. Knopp R, Dailey RH. Central venous cannulation and pressure monitoring. *JACEP* 1977;6:358–366.

23. Flanagan JP, Gradisar IA, Gross RJ, et al. Air embolus: a lethal complication of subclavian venipuncture. *N Engl J Med* 1969;281:488–489.

24. Yeakel AE. Lethal air embolism from plastic blood storage container. *JAMA* 1968;204:267–269.

25. Masoorli S. Managing complications of central venous catheters. *Nursing* 1997;27:59–53.

26. Ducatman BS, McMichan JC, Edwards WD. Catheters-induced lesions of the right side of the heart. A one-year prospective study of 141 autopsies. *JAMA* 1985;253:791–795.

27. Rowley KM, Clubb KS, Smith GJ, et al. Right-sided infective endocarditis as a consequence of flow-directed pulmonary-artery catheterization. A clinicopathologic study of 55 autopsied patients. *N Engl J Med* 1984;311:1152–1156.

28. Conces DJ, Holden RW. Aberrant location and complications in initial placement of subclavian vein catheters. *Arch Surg* 1984;119:293–295.

29. Page AC, Evans RA, Kaczmarski R, Mufti GJ, et al. The insertion of chronic indwelling central venous catheters (Hickman Lines) in interventional radiology suites. *Clin Radiol* 1990;42:105–109.

30. Rasuli P, Hammond DI, Peterkin IR. Spontaneous intra-jugular migration of long-term central venous access catheters. *Radiology* 1992;182:822–824.

31. Defalque RJ, Campbell G. Cardiac tamponade from central venous catheters. *Anesthesiology* 1979;50:249–252.

32. Ellis LM, Vogel SB, Copeland EM. Central venous catheter vascular erosions: diagnosis and clinical course. *Ann Surg* 1989;209:475–478.

33. Henzel JH, DeWeese MS. Morbid and mortal complications associated with prolonged central venous cannulation. *Am J Surg* 1971;121:600–605.

34. Krog M, Berggren L, Brodin M, et al. Pericardial tamponade caused by central venous catheters. *World J Surg* 1982;6:138–143.

35. Stuart RK, Shikora SA, Akerman P, et al. Incidence of arrhythmias with central venous insertion and exchange. *J Parenter Enter Nutr* 1990;14:152–155.

36. Urbaneja A, Fontaine AB, Bruckner M, et al. Evulsion of a Vena Tech filter during insertion of a central venous catheter. *J Vasc Intervent Radiol* 1994;5:783–785.

37. Kaufman JA, Thomas JW, Geller SC, et al. Guide-wire entrapment by inferior vena cava filters: *in vivo* evaluation. *Radiology* 1996;198:71–76.

38. Fan CM. Tunneled catheters. *Semin Intervent Radiol* 1998;15:273–286.

39. Foely MJ. Radiologic placement of long-term central venous access ports: results of 150 patients. *JVIR* 1995;6:255–262.

40. Ahmad I, Ray CE. Radiologic placement of venous access ports. *Semin Intervent Radiol* 1998;15:259–272.

41. Schillinger F, Schillinger D, Montagnac R, et al. Central venous stenosis in hemodialysis: comparative angiographic study of subclavian and internal jugular access. *Nephrologie* 1994;15:129–131.

42. Cimochowski GE, Worley E, Rutherford WE, et al. Superiority of the internal jugular over the subclavian access for temporary dialysis. *Nephron* 1990;54:154–161.

43. Schwab S, Besarab A, Beathard G, et al. *NKF-DOQI clinical practice guidelines for vascular access.* New York: National Kidney Foundation, 1997.

44. Moss JF, Wagman LD, Riihimaki DU, et al. Central venous thrombosis related to silastic Hickman/Broviac catheter in oncologic population. *J Parenter Enter Nutr* 1989;13:397–400.

45. Haire WD, Lieberman P, Lund G, et al. Obstructed central venous catheters: restoring function with 12 hours infusion of urokinase. *Cancer* 1990;66:2279–2285.

46. Bern MM, Lokich JJ, Walach SR, et al. Very low dose of warfarin can prevent thrombosis can prevent central venous catheters: randomized prospective trials. *Ann Intern Med* 1990;112:423–428.

47. Martin C, Viviand X, Saux P, et al. Upper-extremity deep vein thrombosis after central venous catheterization via the axillary vein. *Critical Care Med* 1999;27:2626–2629.

48. Prandoni P, Polistena P, Bernardi E, et al. Upper-extremity deep vein thrombosis: risk factors, diagnosis, and complications. *Arch Intern Med* 1997;157:57–62.

49. Wiener ES, McGuire P, Stolar CJH, et al. The CCSG prospective study of venous access devices: an analysis of insertion and causes of removal. *J Pediatr Surg* 1992;27:155–164.

50. Simpson KR, Hovsepian DM, Picus D. Interventional radiologic placement of chest wall ports: results and complications in 161 consecutive patients. *JVIR* 1997;8:189–195.

51. Sweed M, Vuenter P, Lucente K, et al. Long term central venous catheters in patients with immune deficiency syndrome. *Am J Infect Control* 1995;23:194–199.

52. Early TF, Gregory RT, Wheeler JR, et al. Increased infection rate in double lumen vs single lumen Hickman catheters in cancer patients. *South Med J* 1990;83:34–36.

53. Flowers RH, Schwenzer KJ, Kopel RF, et al. Efficacy of an attachable subcutaneous cuff for prevention of intravascular catheter-related infection: a randomized controlled trial. *JAMA* 1989;261:878–883.

54. Hinke DH, Zandt-Stanley DA, Goodman LR, et al. Pinch off syndrome: a complication of implantable subclavian venous access devices. *Radiology* 1990;177:353–356.

55. Kim DK, Gottesman MH, Forero A, et al. The CVC removal distress syndrome: an unappreciated complication of central venous catheters removal. *Am Surg* 1998;64:344–347.

Subject Index

Note: Page references for figures are followed by f, and page references for tables are followed by t.

A

Accessory cephalic vein, 11
Accessory hemiazygous vein, 16
Access sites, 29–31
Air embolism, 43–45
AJV, 10
Alcohol
  chest port
    insertion, 65f
American Academy of
     Pediatrics guidelines
  pediatric sedation, 116
Anatomic landmark technique
  vs. imaging, 39–42
  results, 60–61, 60t
Angiography suite, 3
Angiography table, 4, 4t
Anterior jugular vein (AJV), 10
Anterior venous drainage
  diaphragm
    above, 9–13
    below, 13–15
Antibiotics
  prophylaxis, 51–52, 76–77
Arm
  anatomy, 52f
  ports, 69
    orientation, 71f
Arteriovenous fistula (AVF), 87
Arteriovenous graft
  neointimal hyperplasia, 88f
AVF, 87
Axillary vein, 12
Azygous vein, 15
Azygous venous system, 15

B

Bacteremia, 92
Bandnet, 128f
Basilic vein, 11
Benzodiazepine, 76
Brachial vein, 12
Brachiocephalic vein, 13
  obstruction, 17
Bradyarrhythmias, 44

Broviac catheters, 75
  care, 82
  infection, 83
  irrigation, 110t
  troubleshooting, 111t
Budd-Chiari syndrome, 78

C

Candida, 70–71
Candida albicans, 83, 113
Carotid artery, 10f
Catheters, 3–4
  Broviac. *See* Broviac
    catheters
  categories, 58t
  central venous. *See* Central
    venous catheters
  characteristics, 59
  chest ports, 63
  clinical indications, 57–59
  flushes, 113–114
  Groshong. *See* Groshong
    catheters
  hemodialysis. *See*
    Hemodialysis catheters
  Hickman. *See* Hickman
    catheters
  hubs
    care, 106–107
  insertion
    complications, 43–44
  insertion site
    care, 107–113
  irrigation, 110t
  Leonard, 111t
  materials, 59
  midline, 98t–100t
  migration, 71–72, 71f
  peripherally inserted central.
    See Peripherally inserted
    central catheters
  polyurethane, 101f
  positioning
    imaging, 45–46
  silicone, 101f

  temporary, 52t, 60t
  transcollateral, 142f
  tunneled. *See* Tunneled
    catheters
  types, 57–59
  ultrasonographically-guided
    placement results, 61t
Cathlink system, 107
CCA
  US, 79
Cefazolin, 52
Central conduit disease
  venographic findings
    risk factors, 36t
Central line
  chest radiography, 45f
Central venous access (CVA)
  contrast computed tomogram,
    27f
  cost analysis, 145–148
  imaging guidance, 19–46
  traditional methods, 26–29
Central venous catheter (CVC)
  defined, 95
Central venous catheter
    placement, 129–143
  alternative techniques,
    131–143
    occluded vein
      recanalization, 131–134
  collateral veins, 143–145
  femoral vein
    CVC catheterization,
      138–141, 139f, 140f,
      141f
  inferior vena cava
    transhepatic
      catheterization, 137–138,
      137t
    translumbar catheterization,
      134–137, 134t
  occlusion prevention,
    130–131
  patient evaluation, 129–130,
    130t

Central venous ports, 63–72
Cephalic vein, 11
Charges
  vs. cost, 146
Chest
  venous anatomy, 12–13
Chest ports, 63–72
  access routes, 65
  catheters, 63
  components, 64f
  design, 63–64
  examples, 64f
  insertion, 65–69
    access establishment, 66
    assembly and implantation,
      66–67
    incision closure, 69
    operator preparation, 66
    patient preparation, 65–66
    pocket creation, 66
    postprocedural
      management, 69
    removal, 69
    skin site preparation, 66
  lumens, 64–65
  outcomes, 69–70
  placement, 67f–68f
  selection, 64–65
  size, 65
Children
  implantable ports, 125f
  PICC, 124f
  VAD placement, 115–128
    clinical situations,
      125–126
    devices, 123–125
    peripheral venous access,
      118–121
    postprocedure care,
      126–128
    sedation, 115–118
    tunneled, 121–123
Collateral veins
  CVC placement, 143–145
  drainage, 16–18
Common carotid artery (CCA)
  US, 79
Contrast computed tomography,
  25
Contrast venography, 22–25
Cost analysis
  CVA, 145–148
  terminology, 145–146

Costs
  vs. charges, 146
  medical procedures, 146t
  streamlining, 146–147
  VAD
    radiologic *vs.* surgical
      placement, 147
CVA. *See* Central venous access
CVC
  defined, 95
Cystic fibrosis, 126

D
Deep sedation, 116
Deep veins
  forearm, 11–12
Devices
  characteristics, 52t
  selection, 49
Dialysis Outcome Quality
    Initiative (DOQI), 58, 92
DOQI, 58, 92
Duplicated inferior vena cava,
  15

E
EJV, 10
  cannulation, 28–29
EMLA cream, 116–117
End-stage renal disease (ESRD),
  87
ESRD, 87
External jugular vein (EJV), 10
  cannulation, 28–29

F
Femoral vein
  CVC catheterization,
    138–141, 139f–140f
Fentanyl, 66, 118
Fibrin sheath, 82–83, 91–92
Fixed cost, 145
Fixed indirect cost, 145–146
Fluoroscopy, 43
  with contrast venography,
    33–35
  guidance, 31–33
Forearm
  deep veins, 11–12

G
Gadolinium, 102
Gadopentate, 102

Groin
  venous anatomy, 14f
Groshong catheters, 75, 97
  dual-lumen, 74f
  irrigation, 110t
Groshong tip, 100–101
Groshong valve, 75f
Guidewires, 3–4
  short, 3

H
Hemiazygous vein, 16
Hemodialysis access, 87–92
Hemodialysis catheters
  complications, 91–92
  evolution, 88
  insertion, 90–91
  selection, 89–90
    access site, 89
  types, 89f
Heparin lock, 108t
Hepatic veins, 14
  anatomy, 15f
Hickman catheters, 75
  care, 82
  infection, 83
  troubleshooting, 111t

I
IJV. *See* Internal jugular vein
Iliac venous system, 14
Imaging
  catheters
    positioning, 45–46
    insertion problems, 42–45
  vs. landmark, 39–42
Imaging-guided CVC
    placement
  complications, 61
Implantable devices
  accessing, 107
Implanted ports, 63–72
  blocked, 109t
  blood sampling, 109t
  bolus injection, 108t
  catheter irrigation, 110t
  characteristics, 52t
  children, 125f
  complications, 70–72
  continuous infusion, 109t
  dressing changes, 109t, 111t
  flushing volumes, 108t
  infection, 70–71

post procedural care,
108t–112t
site preparation, 108t
Incision
care, 107–113
Infants
VAD placement
peripheral venous access,
121
Inferior vena cava (IVC), 14
CVC placement
transhepatic, 134–137, 137t
translumbar, 134–137, 134t
interrupted
with azygous continuation,
15
left-sided, 15
MIP, 28f
translumbar catheter, 135f
Internal jugular vein (IJV),
9–10, 37f
cannulation, 27–29
obstruction
MRI, 53f
portacatheter placement, 30f
puncture, 37f
US, 35–38, 79
vs. landmark, 41t
Interrupted inferior vena cava
with azygous continuation, 15
Interventional radiologist
education, 6–7
role, 1–2
Intravenous sedation
children
VAD placement, 117t
IVC. *See* Inferior vena cava

J
Jugular veins, 9, 10f
Jugular venous arch, 10, 10f

K
Ketamine, 117

L
Left-sided inferior vena cava, 15
Left subclavian vein
hemodialysis, 25f
catheter, 41f
Leonard catheter
troubleshooting, 111t
Lidocaine, 116

Lower extremities
venous drainage, 13–15

M
Magnetic resonance imaging
venography, 25–26
May-Thurner syndrome, 14
Medical procedures
cost, 146t
Metabolic acidosis, 52–53
Microaccess systems, 3–4
Midazolam, 66, 117
Midline catheters, 98t–100t

N
Neck
venous anatomy, 9–10
venous drainage, 17f
Nitroglycerin, 103

O
Occluded superior vena cava
CT, 130f
Occluded veins
recanalization, 131–134
Oral hypoglycemic medication,
52

P
Pain
procedure
clinical signs, 106t
Patients
preparation, 59–60
chest port insertion, 65–66
sterile, 4, 5t
recruitment, 5–6
scheduling, 4–5
Peel-away sheaths, 3
Peripherally inserted central
catheters (PICCs),
95–104, 98t–100t
characteristics, 52t
children, 124f
complications, 102–103, 103t
contraindications, 96–97, 96f
indications, 96, 96f
placement, 101–102
preprocedure preparation, 97
qualifications, 95
terminology, 95
type, 97–101
venous anatomy, 95

Peripheral veins
US, 38–39
Physical examination, 51
Piccline
contrast venography, 33f
PICCs. *See* Peripherally inserted
central catheters
Pinch-off syndrome, 29f
Polyurethane catheters, 101f
Portacaths, 63–72
Ports
arm, 61, 70f
central venous, 63–72
chest. *See* Chest ports
implanted. *See* Implanted
ports
Posterior cardinal veins, 15
Posterior venous drainage,
15–16
Preprocedural assessment,
49–55, 59t
Prilocaine, 116
Procedural review, 20, 20t
Procedure
pain
clinical signs, 106t
Pseudomonas, 83

R
Radically-placed venous access
device
advantages, 2t
Radiologist
education, 6–7
role, 1–2
Rectal carcinoma
chest portacatheter, 40f
Relative value units (RVUs), 146
Right arm
venography, 26f
Right brachiocephalic vein
obstruction, 17f
Right internal jugular vein
hemodialysis, 24f
transverse US, 21f
Right subclavian vein
catheter
hematoma, 39f
fluoroscopic puncture,
32f
sagittal view, 22f, 23f
RVUs, 146

S

Sacrocardinal vein, 15
Saline lock, 108t
Saphenous vein, 13
Sedation
  deep, 116
  pediatric patients
    central VAD placement,
      115–118
Sheath
  fibrin, 82–83, 91–92
  kinking, 43, 44f
  peel-away, 3
Short guidewires, 3
Silicone catheters, 101f
Staphylococcus aureus, 70–71,
  83
Staphylococcus epidermidis,
  70–71, 83
StatLock PICC, 127f
Stenoses
  range, 36t
Subclavian vein, 12–13, 12f
  cannulation, 29
  location, 31f
  obstruction, 18
  stenosis
    angioplasty, 132f
  US, 38, 38f
Subcutaneous tunnel, 79,
  79f–80f
Superior vena cava (SVC),
  13
  fluoroscopy, 42f
  obstruction, 16f, 17
Supracardinal veins, 15
Supraclavicular area
  arterial/venous relationships,
    53f
SVC, 13
  fluoroscopy, 42f
  obstruction, 16f, 17

T

Tachyarrhythmias, 44
Temporary catheters
  characteristics, 52t
  image-guided placement
    indications, 60t
Tissue plasminogen activator
  (TPA), 83, 92
TPA, 83, 92
Transcollateral catheter, 142f
Tunneled catheters, 73–84
  complications, 82–84
  dialysis
    abnormal course,
      50f–51f
  external
    characteristics, 52t
  hemodialysis, 90t
  insertion, 77–81
  postprocedural
    considerations, 77–78
  preprocedural considerations,
    75–77
Twiddler's syndrome, 72

U

Ultrasonographically-guided
  catheter placement
  results, 61t
Ultrasonography (US), 21–22,
  35–39
Upper extremities
  venous anatomy, 10–12
  venous drainage, 11f, 17f
US, 21–22, 35–39

V

VAD. *See* Venous access device
Vancomycin, 77
Variable direct cost, 145
Veins
  anatomy, 9–18

chest, 12–13
  groin, 14f
  neck, 9–10
  PICC, 95–96
  upper extremities,
    10–12
  entry site
    selection, 53–54
  occlusion
    poor catheter tip position,
      131f
Venipuncture, 79
Venography
  contrast, 22–25
Venospasm, 118–121
Venous access device (VAD)
  complications, 151–163
    preoperative assessment,
      151–152
  placement in children,
    115–128
    clinical situations,
      125–126
    devices, 123–125
    peripheral venous access,
      118–121
    postprocedure care,
      126–128
    sedation, 115–118
    tunneled, 121–123
  procedure care, 105–114
    immediate, 106
    long-term, 106–113
  radiologic *vs.* surgical
    placement
    costs, 147
  service, 1–7
    initiation, 5–7
Versed, 76, 117, 118

X

Xylocaine, 66